BUILD STRONG

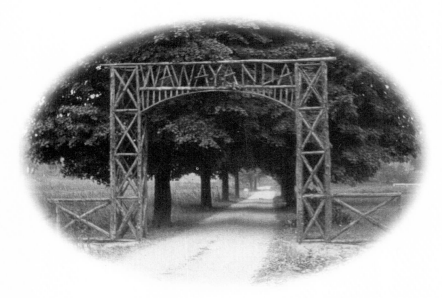

You Can Always Trust
the Great Guide
on the Long Trail

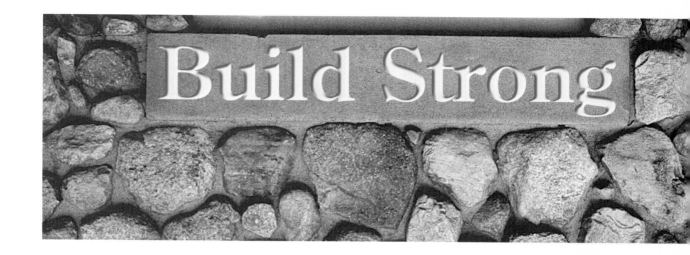

The history of
Camp Wawayanda/Frost Valley YMCA

100 years of building strong kids,
strong families and strong communities

by Diane Galusha

Andy Komonchak, Designer

THE FROST VALLEY YMCA PRESS

Build Strong!

Build Strong!
We must be steady, brave and true.
We must make well all things we do.
Build Strong!

Build Strong!
We must with skill our work endow.
We must not dare to falter now.
Build Strong!

Build Strong!
And when the task is done you'll find,
The product of a thinking mind.
Is Strong!

Frederick Cook 1928

Author: Diane Galusha
Book design: Andy Komonchak

ISBN 0-9675828-4-9

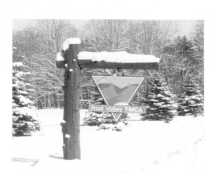

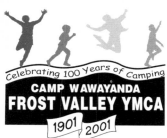

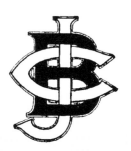

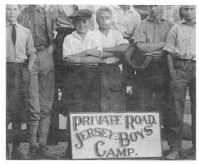

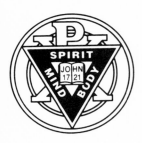

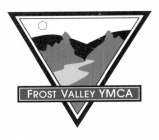

OUR MISSION

**The Frost Valley YMCA
puts Christian principles into practice
through year-round programs
that promote a healthy
spirit, mind and body for all.**

*Consistent with this mission, the Frost Valley YMCA embraces the
guiding principles for developing character: honesty, caring, respect and
responsibility, and seeks to help all people:*

* Develop self-confidence, self-respect and an appreciation for
one's own worth.

* Respect and appreciate the diversity of all human kind.

* Promote the creation of partnerships that support positive
change in our own communities and throughout the world.

* Develop an appreciation for the natural environment and a
commitment to stewardship of the earth's finite resources.

* Visualize a positive future and develop the initiative and
leadership necessary to accomplish this vision.

* Celebrate the cultural and natural heritage of the Catskills,
encouraging opportunities that will cultivate a sense of place.

* Sustain one's spirit, mind and body in an atmosphere that fosters
universal understanding guided by the YMCA's Judeo-Christian
heritage of caring, respect, honesty and responsibility.

Table of Contents

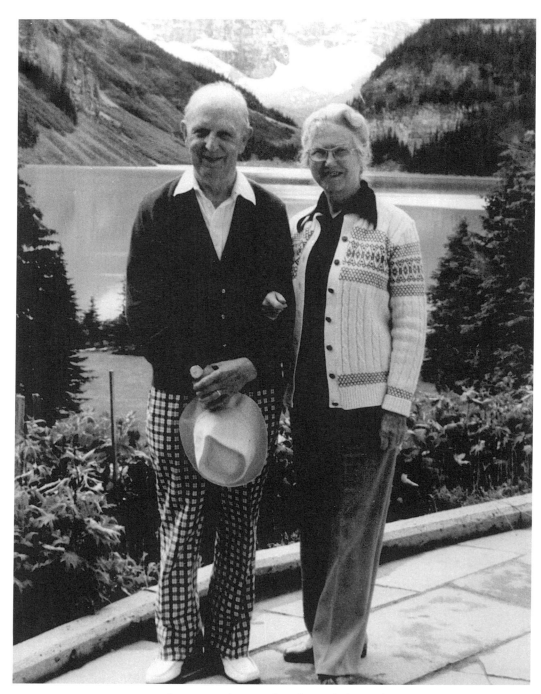

Edmund and Elsie Tomb

DEDICATION

This book is dedicated to the memory of Edmund R. Tomb and his wife, Elsie Tomb. It was their dream to see a history of Camp Wawayanda and the Frost Valley YMCA written and published. Their contribution toward this project, made years ago, has helped to make their dream a reality.

The towering spirit and influence of Edmund R. Tomb and his unyielding determination gave birth and decision to the life of Frost Valley YMCA. The Edmund R. Tomb Administration Building is also dedicated to celebrating his towering spirit and influence. But more than that, during his years with the YMCA, his energy, passion, and vision made a contribution to this movement of monumental proportions. He inspired and empowered, in a very special way, each life he touched. This gentleman was a beacon whose light shone brilliantly, illuminating the way for others to follow.

ACKNOWLEDGMENTS

This book was a joy to write.

It was great fun perusing the many boxes of papers, photographs and artifacts in the Frost Valley archives, pulling together the sturdy threads of an institutional history rich with human drama and delight.

It has been an inspiration, recording a century of challenge, change and social evolution for an organization that has yet remained true to its core mission, that of providing a moral compass for each new generation.

And it has been a privilege to meet so many wonderful individuals who gave freely of their time and memories to help me understand the impact of this place on their lives. Some I have met face to face, some over the telephone, a few I know only through the miracle of e-mail. To all of them I am indebted for their patience, cooperation and amazingly fresh reminiscences.

Special thanks go to Halbe Brown for giving me free access to the wonderfully organized archives and to his invaluable store of personal memories; to Carol O'Beirne for coordinating this important project in all its maddening detail, remaining good-natured throughout; and to Andy Komonchak whose beautiful design created a book that does Frost Valley proud.

I am grateful for the guidance of Frost Valley Alumni Association founder Al Filreis, who provided valuable information, reviewed the manuscript and put me in touch with several other former campers and staff members eager to share their memories.

Former directors, staff members and campers consulted for this project included Earl Armstrong, Leslie Black, Dick Carey, Al Chrone, Bill Devlin, Barry Glickman, Marie Hess, Ted Jackson, Chris Jones, Mike Ketcham, John and Jody Davies Ketcham, Dave and Shirley King, Marie Kremer, Marge Kremer McLaughlin, Jim Marion, Terry and Jacqueline Murray, Randy Reed, Ira Sasowsky, Roy Scutro, Stuart Sherman, David Sunshine, Peter and Claudia Swain and Chuck White.

Long-time Frost Valley staff members John Paul Thomas, Bud Cox and John and Kathy Haskin were tremendously helpful.

Board members who graciously gave of their time and insights included Dr. Edward Ambry, Vern Carnahan, Ed and Jim Ewen, Paul Guenther, Ed Hird, Jim Kellogg, Tom Margetts and Steve Roehm. Thanks, too, to Carolyn English, Eva Gottscho and Emiko and Tatsuo Honma.

Sharing information about their family histories as they relate to Frost Valley were Peter and Richard Forstmann, Jean Freestone, Ted and Helen Tison Hilton, Florence Hart and Roger Straus. Thanks to local history source Karl Connell, and to David Carmichael of the YMCA National Archives, Bob Goodman of Wawayanda State Park, Elliott "Rocky" Gott of Kittatinny Valley State Park, Kurt Oelshlager of Presbyterian Camps and Conference, Inc. (N.J.), Willie Schmidt for historical information on Camp Dudley, and to the staff at the Newburgh Free Library.

Frost Valley staff members interviewed in 2000 included Eric Blum, Mike Dean, Bill Delameter, Kris Henker, Liz Horne, Dan Flanagan, Mike Larison, Jeanna Moyer, Herb Van Baren, Dale Price, Lynn Sturgeon and several counselors and CITs whose enthusiasm was infectious but who, alas, remain nameless.

To those who have been inadvertently overlooked, I offer my apologies, and my sincere thanks.

Diane Galusha

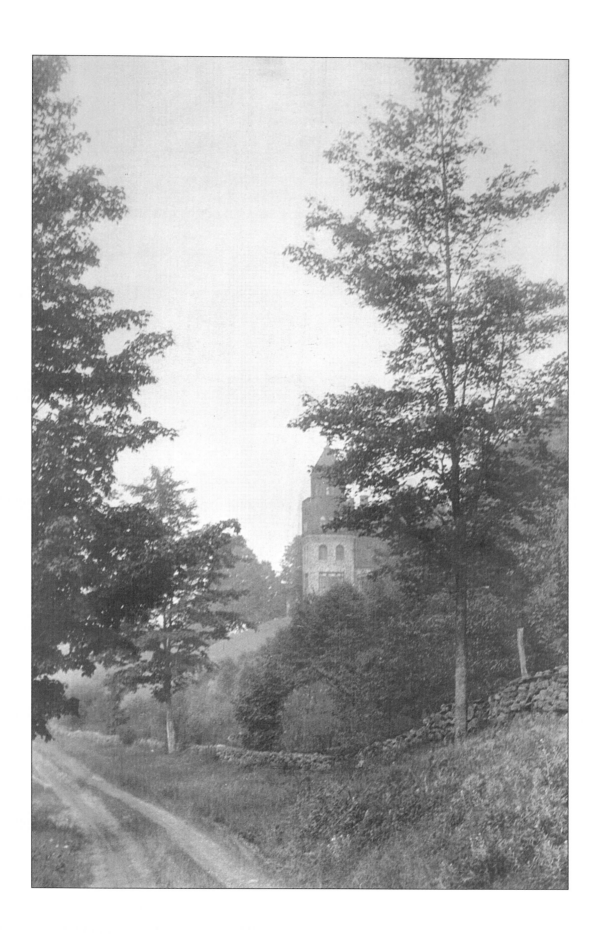

Build Strong

CAMP WAWAYANDA/FROST VALLEY TIME LINE

1885	Wawayanda's beginnings: Newburgh YMCA sponsors teenage camping excursion to Orange Lake, N.Y., led by Sumner Dudley	
	Previous year's experiment repeated at Lake Wawayanda, Sussex County, N.J. and continues each summer for New York and New Jersey YMCA members	**1886**
1891	Lake Wawayanda campsite proves inadequate to the demand; Camp moves to Lake Champlain, N.Y., and is later named Camp Dudley after its founder	
	New Jersey boys return to Lake Wawayanda to attend YMCA camp under Director Charles R. Scott	**1901**
1906	U.S. Volunteer Lifesaving Corps offers first lifesaving instruction at Camp Wawayanda; training methods later adopted by Red Cross	
	Camp Wawayanda hosts training for leaders of the newly established Boy Scouts of America	**1911**
1919	Camp property in Sussex County sold; Wawayanda moves to new site in Andover, N.J.	
	Main lodge at New Camp Wawayanda dedicated to 18 camp alumni killed in World War I	**1920**

1921	C. R. Scott retires as Camp Director	
	John Ledlie begins 15-year Camp Directorship; reorganizes linear camp layout into age-related "villages"	**1930**
1946	Lodge in Outpost Village dedicated to 30 Wawayanda alumni killed in World War II	
	Encroaching development prompts sale of Andover site; C. R. Scott dies	**1954**
1955	Camp Wawayanda spends first of three summers at interim site, Stevens Institute of Technology Camp at Johnsonburg, N.J.	
	A Christmas Eve deal secures YMCA purchase of Julius Forstmann's 2,200-acre estate in the Catskill Mountains of New York	**1956**
1957	Frost Valley Association formed to run the Frost Valley Camp and Conference Center; Forstmann "Castle" opens to families and conference groups	
	First summer camp held at Frost Valley, for boys only	**1958**
1962	Girls camp (later named Camp Henry Hird) opens	
	Halbe Brown begins 35-year tenure as Executive Director of Frost Valley	**1966**

1968	Frost Valley becomes an independent YMCA	FROST VALLEY YMCA
	Environmental Education Center established; dedicated to Woodruff J. English in 1985	**1969**
1975	First-ever dialysis center for campers with kidney ailments opens in partnership with Ruth Carole Gottscho Foundation; 640-acre Tison estate added to Frost Valley as the Alexander Tison Trust Preserve	
	1,600-acre Straus estate acquired; Wellness Program and Curriculum developed	**1978**
1979	Tokyo-New York YMCA Partnership formed	
	Sagendorf Country Museum completed; Thomas Lodge dining hall destroyed by fire on New Year's Eve	**1982**
1983	First Elderhostel Program at Frost Valley; Camps Wawayanda for Boys and Hird for Girls transformed into co-educational, age-based camps	
	Acid rain research program begins with U. S. Geological Survey; Mainstreaming at Camp (MAC) launched for children with developmental disabilities	**1984**
1985	YMCA Camping Centennial celebrated	
	Dedication of reconstructed Thomas Lodge	**1986**

1988	Forest Management Trail developed; Raptor Center and Wildlife Rehabilitation Program established	
	Resource Management Compost Center and Greenhouse becomes operational; three new lodges open, replacing cabin groups	1990
1992	Ketcham Chapel and Memorial Garden dedicated	
	Dedication of Edmund R. Tomb Administration Building and Historical Center	1993
1995	Hayden Observatory opens	
	Dedication of Tokyo-Frost Valley Friendship House	1996
1998	Dedication of USGS-Frost Valley Streamside Classroom; Luke Roehm Technology Learning Center opens	
	Frost Valley Community Center opens, providing After-School Child Care and Summer Day Camp for area children	1999
2000	Frost Valley Farm established; major Castle restoration project begins	
	Wawayanda-Frost Valley Centennial celebrated	2001

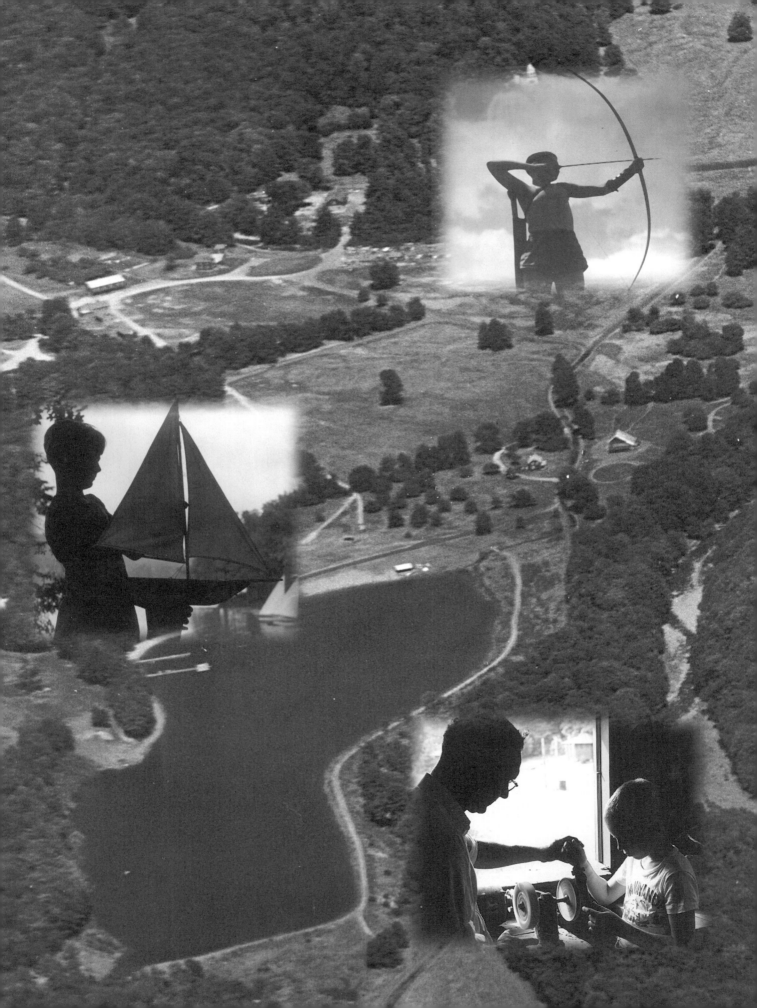

Prologue

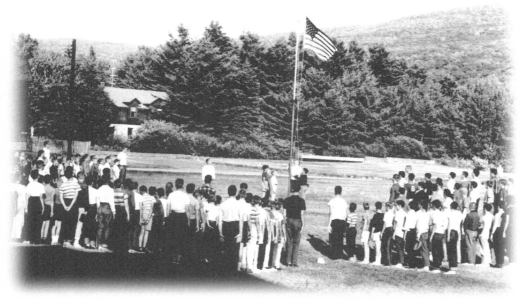

It is a fine morning in late June, the kind that pushes the snows of a Catskill winter, and the recent cold rains of spring, into the dim corners of memory. A light breeze propels puffy white clouds across an azure sky. The mountains are a deep, deep green, made lustrous by an overnight shower that has added energy to an already-rollicking Biscuit Brook.

It is an ideal day to start the Summer 2000 camping season at Frost Valley YMCA. Mother Nature has pulled out all the stops to welcome 427 girls and boys who will spend at least the next two weeks in her domain. Returning campers know that Mother's fickle disposition may make the valley a different place tomorrow; indeed, a booming thunderstorm that rattles the cabin rooftops this night will make Catskill weather "veterans" out of first-timers, too.

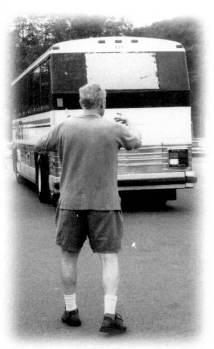

But that's a few hours into the future. Right now, there is electricity enough on the broad grassy field, where parents, campers and siblings are unloading car trunks; in the administration building parking lot where the first of five buses from Montclair and Teaneck and Newark and New York City delivers 40 young passengers into the sunshine; and beneath the big striped tent where a small army of red-shirted Counselors-in-Training heft duffel bags and backpacks, guitars and bicycles onto trucks bound for hillside cabin villages.

Excitement permeates the place. There are joyful shrieks as former campmates see each other for the first time in a year, and happy shouts as they learn they will share a cabin again. For some, words are not needed to convey delight. An eight-year-old named Carlos fairly leaps off the bus, runs happily across 20 feet of parking lot to bestow a hearty hug on Malcolm Sadler, who, surprised, nevertheless returns the hug and Carlos' wide smile. The two have never met, but they have one thing in common. They are both first-timers – Carlos in the Mainstreaming at Camp (MAC) program for developmentally disabled youngsters, and Malcolm as a counselor for Phoenix Camp, a month-long leadership program for 15-year-olds.

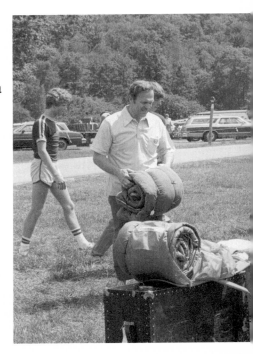

For Halbe Brown, Frost Valley's Executive Director who has been on hand for the first day of camp every summer since 1966, this day has a familiar feel. With the practiced air of an experienced traffic cop, Halbe directs bus driver Joe Warren to the proper unloading spot, then sets to work grabbing trunks and bags from the bus' baggage compartment. He wipes sweat from his brow, and wears an expression of pure pleasure.

So does Lexi Cariello, 13, of Maplewood, N.J. She and Danielle Rem, also 13, of Teaneck, are here for their sixth year of swimming and hiking, campfires and challenge nights. How to articulate the Frost Valley appeal? "You end up making a family here," explains Lexi. "There's a strong sense of knowing who you are." And who your friends are. Lexi and Danielle say they'll be firm friends forever.

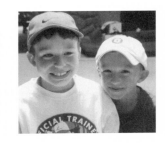

Such relationships are forged and nourished as campers discover shared interests, or experience new activities and challenges together. It may be archery, woodworking, soccer or astronomy; horseback riding, environmental study, painting or poetry. Want to experience high adventure? The list of camp-sponsored trips this year includes sailing on Lake George, rafting in North Carolina, or biking along the coast of the Pacific Northwest.

Nor are children with special needs excluded from the fun. In addition to the MAC program, children with kidney ailments get the chance to go to camp because Frost Valley has a dialysis center with a specially-trained medical staff.

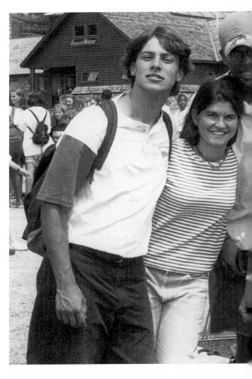

Much of what Frost Valley camping is today would be unrecognizable to the founders of its parent camp, Wawayanda, which was officially launched a century ago on the northern New Jersey lake of that name. Then, as the YMCA's New Jersey Boys Camp, it was open to males only. It featured activities like model boat building, knot tying, and signaling, but had a decidedly religious flavor, with Bible study, evening vespers and hymn sings important aspects of the program. Boys were supervised by adult volunteers who were considered to be in good Christian standing. They slept in tents, enjoyed stereopticon lectures and competed for certificates which rewarded their knowledge of the natural world.

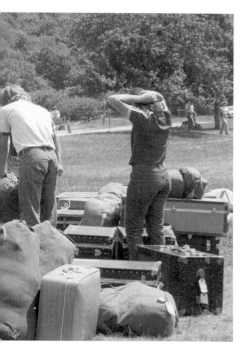

Over the years, the activities and atmosphere at camp reflected changing interests and societal influences. When radio began to entertain awestruck listeners, Wawayanda installed a "radiotelephone" to provide baseball scores and concerts from as far away as Boston and Schenectady. When Charles Lindbergh flew solo across the Atlantic, interest soared in model airplane building at camp. When World War II patriotism gripped the nation, Wawayanda campers were taught the "Three Rs of Wartime Camping: Resourcefulness, Responsibility and Ruggedness."

In 1962, girls were welcomed into the camp population, signaling a move toward the inclusiveness that would, in coming decades, reflect the addition of all races, ethnic groups and nationalities in the complexion of Frost Valley. In the 1980s, new emphasis was placed on physical and emotional well-being, personal fitness and balance. Encouraging the adoption of ethical values replaced overt evangelism in a more ecumenical camp atmosphere.

Frost Valley has become much more than a summer camp, of course. It is an important center for environmental education and research. It is a conference center offering a stimulating environment for meetings and seminars. It is a year-round recreation and cultural center for families, youth groups and senior citizens. Its partnership with the Tokyo YMCA offers a forum for international exchange, understanding and appreciation.

But at Frost Valley's core, at the heart of its history, is summer camp: swimming lessons, village cheers in the dining hall, singing "Wawayanda Grace," listening to the unfamiliar sounds of a forest night, letters from home, fireside conversations with cabin-mates and counselors who have become friends. And at the root of YMCA summer camp are values that over the decades have changed only in some respects. Wawayanda's first director, Charles R. Scott, articulated those values as "Order, Cleanliness, Respect and Service to Others." Today's YMCA programs emphasize "Respect, Caring, Honesty and Responsibility."

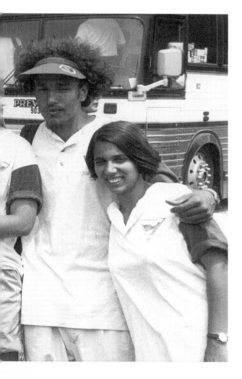

Those values are what drew Felicity and Paul Kelcourse to Frost Valley as counselors in 1977, and brought them back in 2000 to give daughter Rosalinde her first summer camp experience. When they met 23 years ago, it was as leaders of a Frost Valley teen adventure trip from Alberta, Canada, to New Mexico. For five weeks they shepherded a group of teenagers on a 5,000-mile journey that included backpacking and whitewater rafting in the rugged Rockies. They survived physical challenges, health emergencies and all manner of foul weather. "And we still got married," laughs Felicity. She is now a professor at a Quaker seminary in Indianapolis; her husband is a Quaker pastor.

Back then, they say, they didn't care about their counselor's pay; it was the doing, and the learning, that were important. As it turns out, Felicity says, "It was good training for life."

The Kelcourses have returned to Frost Valley to give their daughter the sense of belonging that is unique to this special extended community. Indeed, there is a common bond between Frost Valley campers, staff members and volunteers. Once you become a member of the Frost Valley family, you are always welcomed home.

And so the Kelcourses found themselves on a camp path this beautiful June day, chatting with Halbe Brown about Frost Valley, about what's new . . . and what isn't . . . in the valley of the Neversink. Brown, who would retire after one more year at the helm of this diversified, wide-reaching institution, pointed forward, to the fledgling demonstration farm where sustainable agricultural practices will be the focus; to the envisioned semester-long program for environmental study; to the less visionary, but nonetheless necessary, task of erecting a pavilion as a staging area for crowded camp registration days such as these.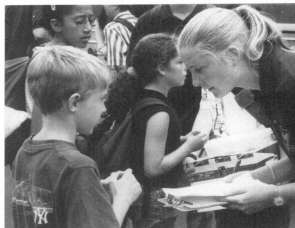

The Kelcourses listen with genuine interest to all of these projections for the future. And then, taking in the wide valley, the sparkling lake, the cool and fragrant woods beside the path, Felicity says, "Well, it's nice to come back and see the place hasn't changed that much."

No, it is still a great place to spend a few golden weeks of summer when you are young and the world awaits. Charles R. Scott may have been talking about Frost Valley and its mission as he wrote 50 years ago, "When we think of youth, we usually think of physical vigor, their interest in athletics and in social activities, but we must not forget that this is also the age for dreaming dreams, seeing visions and a time of great imagination and ideals."

Encouraging young people and their dreams motivated Wawayanda's founders. It continues to guide the committed leaders of Frost Valley.

Some things, you might say, never change.

Beginnings. The Young Men's Christian Association was founded June 6, 1844 in London by George Williams, a 23-year-old store clerk, who, with several other young men, had come together around Bible study and prayer. The YMCA's membership expanded as young males found it an antidote to long hours, difficult working conditions and squalid urban life. George Williams was knighted by Queen Victoria in 1894 for his YMCA work.

• *The Movement Spreads.* The YMCA was established in North America (Montreal and Boston) in 1851. By 1854, branches were formed in several cities across the U.S., including Jersey City, New Brunswick and Newark, N.J. The first International Y Conference was held in Paris in 1855, drawing representatives from 329 YMCAs in nine nations, with 30,360 members.

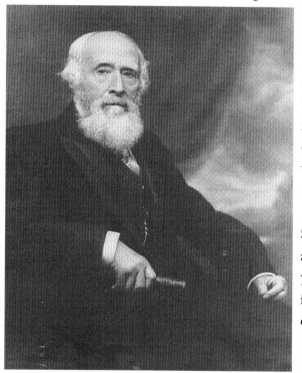

Sir George Williams, founder of the YMCA

• *Y Work.* The Y became known for conducting Sunday Schools and religious mission work, for helping the destitute and for providing room, board and employment assistance to young men newly arrived or adrift in the city. Libraries, reading rooms, gymnasiums and interdenominational lectures and classes later became Y hallmarks.

• *War Work.* During the Civil War, the Y spurred volunteer efforts to help soldiers and prisoners of war, and to distribute a million Bibles. Three generations later, the Y raised millions of dollars and hired thousands of men and women to run military canteens and post exchanges to assist soldiers in World War I. Later, during World War II, the YMCA was a major player in the United Service Organization – USO – a coalition of agencies formed to provide social outlets and recreation for servicemen and women. YMCAs also worked with interned Japanese Americans.

• *Springfield College.* The School for Christian Workers, later known as the International YMCA Training School, and finally as Springfield College, was established in 1885 in Springfield, Mass. to train lay religious workers, including YMCA secretaries. In 1891,

Luther Gulick, a physician and physical education instructor at Springfield, developed the YMCA's now-familiar inverted red triangle to symbolize "man's essential unity: body, mind and spirit. . . a wonderful combination of the dust of the earth and the breath of God." Springfield was the first of 20 YMCA-affiliated colleges to be established by 1950. Unlike most of the others, Springfield remains firmly linked to the movement.

• *Camping.* In 1885, Sumner Dudley, at the request of Newburgh YMCA Secretary George A. Sanford, took seven teenagers on a week-long camping excursion to Orange Lake near Newburgh, N.Y. While not the first recorded camping trip conducted by a Y, Dudley's experiment led to the establishment of Camps Wawayanda and Dudley, and spawned the summer camp movement in the U.S. This also marked a period of increased attention by the YMCA to the needs of boys, as well as young men.

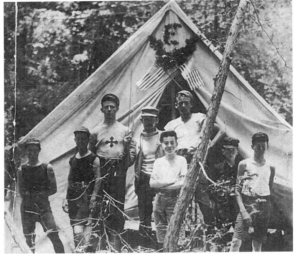

7 boys camping at Orange Lake, Newburgh, N.Y. began the summer camp movement in the United States.

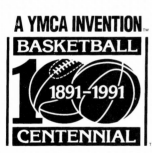

A YMCA INVENTION

BASKETBALL

100

1891–1991

CENTENNIAL

• *Athletic Firsts.* In 1891, James Naismith, an instructor at Springfield College, developed the game of basketball as an indoor substitute for football. The game proved wildly popular and spread across the country after its description and rules were published in *The Triangle* magazine in January, 1892. Volleyball (initially called "mintonette") was invented at the Holyoke, Mass. YMCA by William G. Morgan. The YMCA's Camp Wawayanda was among the first to offer lifesaving and swimming safety instruction, and a Springfield College student, George Goss, wrote the first American book on lifesaving in 1913 as a thesis. A YMCA official encouraged the Red Cross to include lifesaving instruction in its disaster and wartime services programs. The YMCA Swimming and Lifesaving Manual (1919) was one of the earliest works on the sub-

James Naismith, the inventor of the game of basketball, and his wife, the former Maude Sherman, standing next to some of the original equipment.

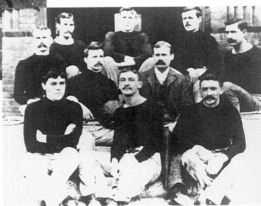

The First Basketball Team-1891
These 9 players played 9 classmates in the first Basketball game while attending the International YMCA Training School (Springfield College).

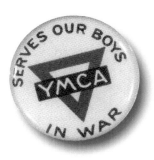

ject. The game of racquetball was invented in 1950 at the Greenwich, Conn. YMCA by member George Sobek.

• *John R. Mott.* A beacon for the YMCA's international work was John R. Mott, the Methodist evangelist who was born in Livingston Manor, Sullivan County, N.Y. in 1865. A founder, in 1895, of the World's Student Christian Federation, he served as president of the World Alliance of YMCAs from 1926 to 1937, and of the International Missionary Council from 1921 to 1942. He was awarded the Nobel Peace Prize in 1946 for his efforts to promote interdenominational cooperation among Christians.

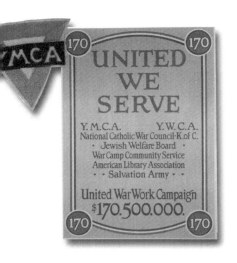

• *Depression Work.* During the Great Depression of the 1930s, YMCAs provided free medical services, physical programs, school classes and social outlets for unemployed young men. Ys built partnerships with other social welfare agencies to respond to increased demand and dwindling resources.

• *Family Focus.* Emphasis gradually shifted toward youth and families. More and more Ys admitted women, and following the post-war trend, many extended their operations to the suburbs.

• *Reassessment.* Following the unrest, apathy and disenchantment of the 1960s and early 1970s, the YMCA reassessed its mission and goals, renewed its outreach efforts, and responded to individual community needs with health and fitness programming, child care, substance abuse prevention, job training, family activities and specialized camping for distinct audiences.

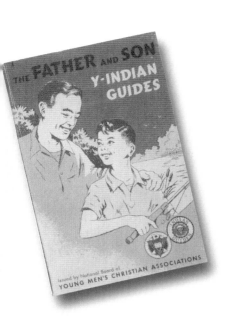

And, harkening back to its roots, the Y placed new emphasis on character development, specifying four "core values" – caring, honesty, respect and responsibility. These values are woven into YMCA programs and form the backbone of a movement that in 2001, the year of its 150th anniversary, serves nearly 17 million Americans and 30 million more around the world.

Sources: History of the YMCA in North America, by C. Howard Hopkins, Association Press, NY, 1951; John R. Mott, 1865-1955, A Biography by C. Howard Hopkins, William B. Eerdmans Publishing Co., Grand Rapids, 1979; YMCA Camping, An Abbreviated History, by Eugene A. Turner, Jr., YMCA of the USA, 1984; and the YMCA of the USA web site: www.ymca.net.

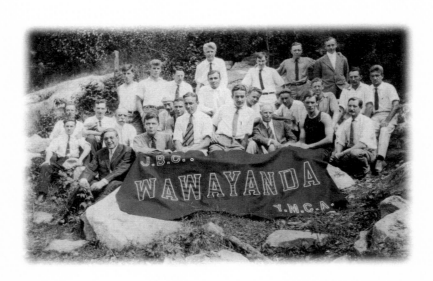

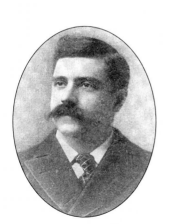

Sumner F. Dudley

"Never attempt any work with boys except it tends permanently to advance the Kingdom of God."
Sumner Dudley

He wasn't the biggest man George Peck had ever known, but when it came to what really mattered – compassion, strength of character, and leadership – Sumner Francis Dudley had no equal.

"He was a man of most pleasing personality, possessing a manner that easily and naturally attracted men as well as boys," Mr. Peck would later write of the man he most admired. Handsome, strong and a terrific swimmer, Sumner Dudley boasted a barrel chest and a big heart to fill it. "He quickly made friends by his willingness and desire to help any who needed counsel and advice," recalled Mr. Peck. "No sacrifice was ever too great for him."

He might also have been hailed for his pioneering spirit, for Sumner Dudley was the man credited with launching the summer camping movement in the United States by establishing the forerunner of Camp Wawayanda.

The Young Men's Christian Association, begun in London in 1844, had been established in America in 1851 to minister to the spiritual, physical, intellectual and employment needs of young men, those in their late teens and early 20s. While many Ys conducted Sunday Schools for youngsters, or provided food and other relief to destitute children, it wasn't until the 1870s that the movement began to provide organized programs for boys, those 12 to 18 years old. On the theory that adult values are forged in youth, the Y's new Boys Department offered teenagers activities ranging from physical education classes to Bible study.

A New York City businessman, Sumner Dudley was also an active YMCA volunteer, both in New York and New Jersey. In 1883, he organized a boys' literary society at the New York City Y, establishing high standards for debate, reading and parliamentary practice. He advocated involvement of boys in YMCA conferences and regional meetings, and actively consulted these young participants in decisions related to boys work activities. Thus he gained the attention

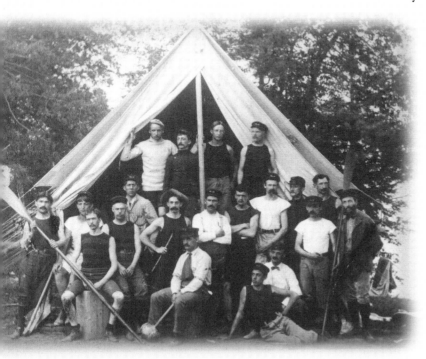

Sumner Dudley [front center with mallet] at first Lake Wawayanda Camp, Sussex County N.J. in 1886.

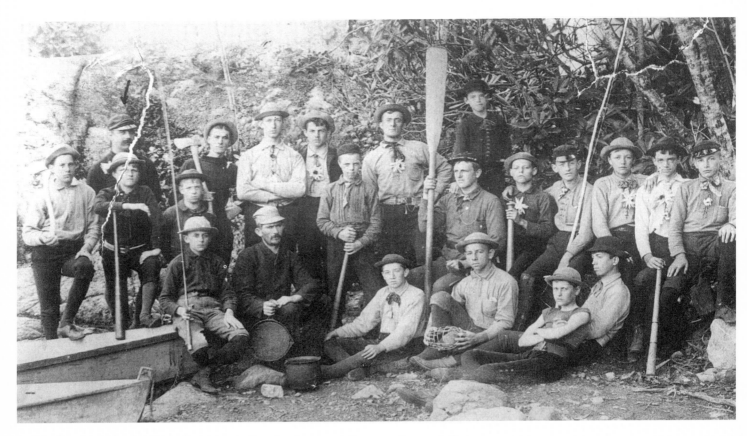

Lake Wawayanda, 1886

of Y leaders, including George A. Sanford, general secretary of the
Newburgh Association, who asked Dudley to organize a one-week
camping excursion for a handful of boys. Sanford suggested his own
school-boy camping grounds at Wawayanda Lake, New Jersey, near
his old home at Warwick, N.Y., however, that first year, 1885, the Y-
sponsored outing was held at Mombasha Lake, now known as
Orange Lake, near Newburgh.

George Peck was among seven teenagers who accompanied
leader Dudley on the initial outing of the "Boys Camping Society"
(BCS) that July. They slept on blankets on the bare ground, and
rowed about the lake in a borrowed boat. "Our equipment was quite
simple," he remembered. "We had one tent in which we lived and
ate our meals in rainy weather. Each camper brought his own table
equipment, and as far as I can recall, our cooking outfit was made up
of one frying pan, two pails and a coffee pot. The meals were prepared over an open fireplace built around stones. We had no table
but in fair weather we ate our meals from a rubber blanket spread
on the ground. Mr. Dudley cooked the meals and the boys washed
the dishes. Our chief pleasures were eating and swimming. We were
unable to indulge in games to any great extent, but we will never forget the daily Bible study and the evening talks around the camp fire

*"We were unable
to indulge in games
to any great extent,
but we will never
forget the daily
Bible study and the
evening talks
around the camp
fire just before
retiring."*

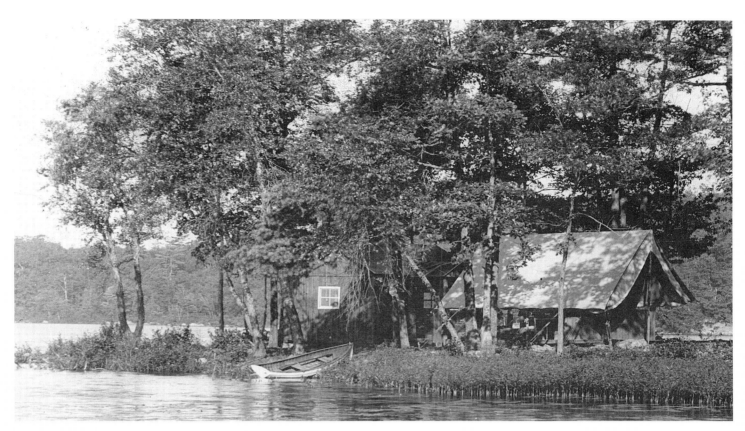

Headquarters of first Wawayanda island campsite. Campers arrived at the campsite after a mile-and-a-half row across Lake Wawayanda.

just before retiring."

Wrote George Sanford in 1920, "The outstanding features were Bible study, testimony and prayer. On the rocks near the lake at the beginning of the day, and in the boat as darkness closed in, we sang and prayed."

Indeed, a knowledge of the Bible was a prerequisite to attend BCS that first year. Prospective campers had to take an admissions test after studying a syllabus of Bible passages and objectives of the YMCA which could be obtained by sending 15 cents to Dudley. Boys had to be at least 14, and have parental permission. The first campers were George Peck, George Weller, D. Bryant Turner, Fred B. Howell, Robert D. Oakley, Isaac Oakley and Frank G. Kimble.

Dudley's subsequent report on the Orange Lake adventure was short on words, but long on enthusiasm: "Weather: delightful . . . Fishing: very moderate. Swimming: called for three times a day. Health: good. Accidents: none. Appetites: ravenous. Hearty, manly fun: any quantity. Good nature: largely developed."

To be sure, this was not the first experiment in summer camping. Other organizations, and YMCAs in Virginia, Michigan and Brooklyn, had conducted similar "camping out" excursions during the 1880s. But Dudley's unique formula for promoting individual spiritual development along with a love of the natural world, was a winning one that contributed to the long-term success of the enterprise.

He recognized that the informal, intimate nature of summer camping and the special group dynamics associated with it could be utilized in developing Christian values and lifestyles. "Pleasure seeking does not necessitate any relaxation of Christian study and work," Dudley said.

Thus, "Camp Baldhead," so nicknamed for the close-cropped haircuts of the campers, was conducted again the following year, this time at Wawayanda Lake, in Sussex County, New Jersey, to accommodate a growing campership.

Twenty-three campers came to Wawayanda from Newburgh, Brooklyn and Newark, and the "camping season" was extended to two weeks. Boys were advised to bring wool or knit stocking caps for sleeping and to protect against insect bites, a suit of winter underwear, flannel shirts, fishing tackle, a baseball glove and a Bible, all to fit in a wooden box two feet by one foot by one foot.

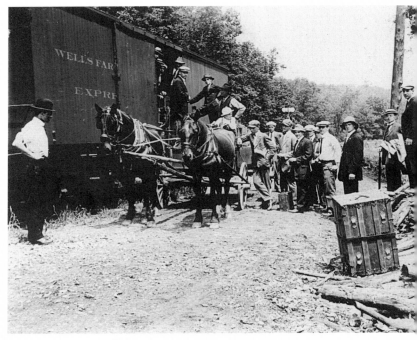

Campers embarking on the 7-mile trip from the train in Warwick, N.Y. to Wawayanda.

They'd have done well to bring foul weather gear to the campsite in 1886. Campers took the train to Warwick, N.Y., then walked seven miles in the driving rain to Wawayanda, where they had to row a mile-and-a-half across the lake to the island where they were to camp. They got one large tent up, then huddled inside eating a supper of rain-soaked bread and cold ham. The boys wrapped themselves in blankets while Dudley spent the night drying sodden clothing by the fire.

The camp occupied this spot in the rolling hills of northern New Jersey for the next four summers. Enrollment reached 35 in 1887. Sixty-five campers enrolled in 1889, when it cost $2.75 to take the train from New York to Warwick, and 75 cents a day for camp board. "A small store near the camp has confectionary, peanuts and soda for sale. Beyond a small allowance for such things, the boys need not to be at any expense other than that stated above," explained the first camp brochure, published in 1889.

In 1888, at age 33, Dudley left the family business, Shepard and

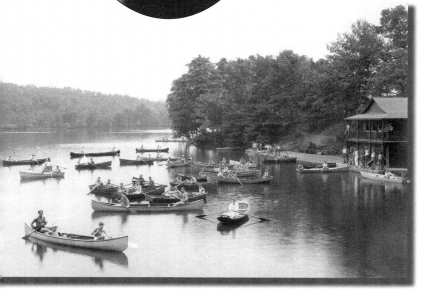

Dudley, manufacturers of surgical instruments, in order to devote full time to YMCA work. He served as general secretary of the Orange N.J. YMCA, then became a member of the Board of Directors. He was also a member of the New Jersey and New York State Committees, and served as first chairman of the New Jersey State Boys Work Committee, all the while directing the summer camp under the auspices of both State Committees.

When, in 1891, the camp outgrew its island home on Lake Wawayanda, Dudley sought out a new location, and found it on Lake Champlain, 300 miles away, on land donated by J. H. Worman, editor of Outing Magazine. For the next ten years, boys from New York and New Jersey spent summer vacations on the big lake. Through growth and change, Dudley remained committed to the camp and its ideals, developing procedures and camp management practices that would influence a growing number of YMCA camps. (By 1905, the YMCA reported that 6,348 boys were enrolled in 187 camps.) He was, above all, confident in the model he had developed.

"The camp is not an experiment," Dudley explained after several years at the helm, "but is founded upon earnest prayer, careful thought and long experience. Everything that is good, pure and jolly is indulged in." He did not mention that he had poured a considerable amount of his own private resources into the enterprise.

The visionary Mr. Dudley left a sturdy legacy when he died of Bright's disease, a kidney ailment, on March 14, 1897 at the age of 43. The camp on the shores of Lake Champlain was afterwards named for him. It would move three more times in the vicinity of Westport, N.Y. before, in 1904, settling at the site it has occupied continuously ever since. Former camper George Peck had the unenviable task of stepping into his mentor's shoes to direct Camp Dudley from 1897 to 1903.

In 1900, when, again, the number of campers – 200 – stretched the limits of the facilities, the New Jersey State YMCA Committee decided to go back "home," to Lake Wawayanda. Enter Charles Richard Scott, a name that would become synonymous with the future Camp Wawayanda.

"The camp is not an experiment," Dudley explained after several years at the helm, "but is founded upon earnest prayer, careful thought and long experience. Everything that is good, pure and jolly is indulged in."

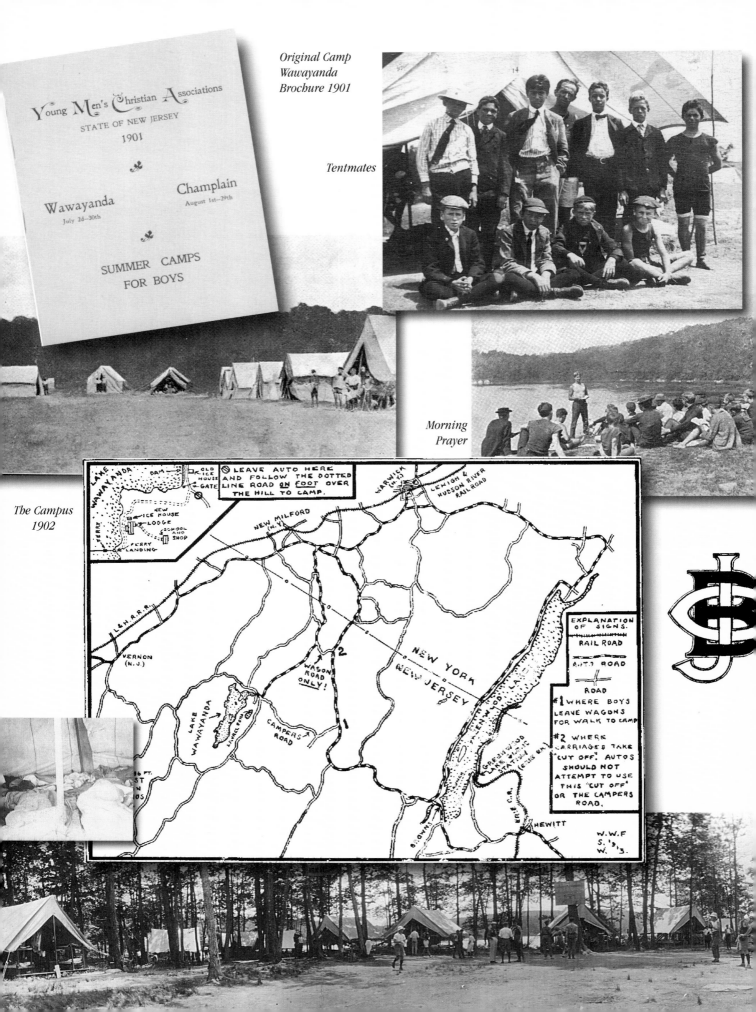

Young Men's Christian Associations
STATE OF NEW JERSEY
1901

Wawayanda
July 2d–30th

Champlain
August 1st–29th

SUMMER CAMPS
FOR BOYS

*Original Camp
Wawayanda
Brochure 1901*

Tentmates

*Morning
Prayer*

*The Campus
1902*

LEAVE AUTO HERE
AND FOLLOW THE DOTTED
LINE ROAD ON FOOT OVER
THE HILL TO CAMP.

LAKE WAWAYANDA
DAM
OLD ICE HOUSE
GATE
FERRY
NEW ICE HOUSE
LODGE
SCHOOL AND SHOP
FERRY LANDING

WARWICK (N.Y.)
LEHIGH & HUDSON RIVER RAILROAD

NEW MILFORD (N.Y.)

VERNON (N.J.)

L&H.R.R.

WAGON
ROAD
ONLY!

LAKE WAWAYANDA

CAMPERS
ROAD

NEW YORK
NEW JERSEY

GREENWOOD LAKE

EXPLANATION
OF SIGNS.
RAIL ROAD
AUTO ROAD
ROAD
#1 WHERE BOYS
LEAVE WAGONS
FOR WALK TO CAMP
#2 WHERE
CARRIAGES TAKE
"CUT OFF". AUTOS
SHOULD NOT
ATTEMPT TO USE
THIS "CUT OFF"
OR THE CAMPERS
ROAD.

HEWITT

W.W.F
S. 1913.
W.

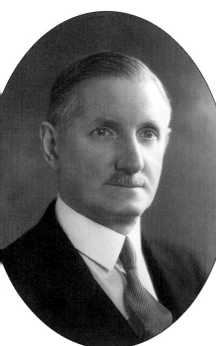

Charles R. Scott

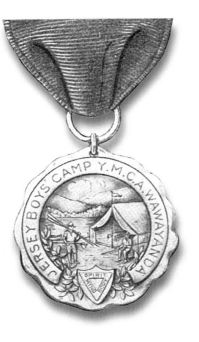

Many a boy is hungry, starving for a little work and love." Charles R. Scott, writing his memoirs as an elderly man, penned that unattributed quote among his "Enduring Memories." He didn't explain why, but it may well have been his rationale for a lifetime in the service of New Jersey youth.

Scott was the YMCA's State Boys Work Secretary for 33 years and Director of the New Jersey Boys Camp – Camp Wawayanda – for 21 of those years. It was his job to organize the return of the camp from Lake Champlain to New Jersey in 1901, and it would be his task to move it again in 1919. With his wife and three children sharing his tent in the Jersey woods, he supervised camp operations every summer, guiding a generation of boys through the Wawayanda passage to find their way in the world. Charles R. Scott lived and breathed the YMCA, and, in fact, passed his last moments surrounded by exhuberant boys in Wawayanda's dining hall on a fine summer day in 1954.

His journey to a career with the Y began in Brooklyn, where, as a youth, he clerked in his parents' cigar and cutlery store, sold newspapers on street corners, and accompanied his cousins as they delivered meat from his uncle's market. When his family faced hard economic times, he left school at age 14 to go to work, finding a job through the help of the Employment Secretary at the 23rd Street Branch of the YMCA. He tried balancing work with architectural classes at night at the New York Mechanics and Tradesmen's School, but had to give up the latter when his health began to suffer.

Moving with his family to Belleville, N.J., Scott joined the Newark YMCA, where he attended gymnasium class, and "learned the drills of dumb bells and Indian clubs." The idea of getting paid to work for the Y appealed to Scott, and he, in turn, impressed Newark Secretary Henry Cozzens, who offered him a job as his assistant. Salary: $8 a week. "I accepted and was 'on trial' for one month beginning October 1, 1893," wrote Scott some years later. "At the close of the month, nothing was said, so I continued 'on trial' until my retirement."

Scott, who was not yet 20, was made Boys Work Secretary for the Newark Y, organizing physical programs, lectures and other activities for fellow teenagers. Among his first tasks was to convert a damp, moldy basement bowling alley at the Clinton Street Y into the "Boys Room." Participation in the programs grew and so did admiration for Scott's abilities.

In 1901, Charles Kilborne, who had succeeded Sumner Dudley as Chairman of the New Jersey Boys Work Committee, tapped Charles R. Scott to become the first New Jersey State Boys Work Secretary. It was a bittersweet time for Scott, as his wife, Mary Philipson Scott, and their infant son both died during childbirth just ten days before he was to start at his new post.

Yet despite his grief, he summoned the will to plunge into the job, and perhaps found some measure of comfort in the demands of

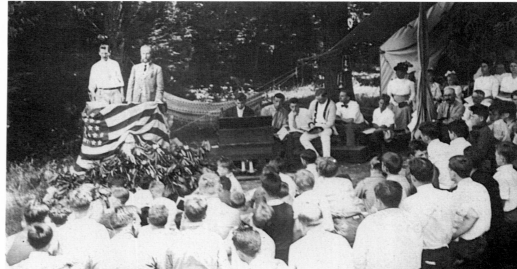

The Jersey Boys Camp logo, shown on Director Charles R. Scott's sweater, above right.

re-establishing a summer camp in New Jersey. The state committee had authorized the move from crowded Camp Dudley on Lake Champlain, and a committee of three men – Oranges Association Secretary Willard Smith, George Hageman and William Janiway – accompanied Scott on a springtime bicycle tour of northern New Jersey in search of a suitable camp site. The group was drawn to Lake Wawayanda where

Charles Kilborne and Charles Scott lead a Wawayanda Sunday prayer service.

Dudley and company had made camp from 1886 to 1891. They arranged a five-year lease with the Fancher family which owned part of the land, and then secured lake privileges from the Thomas Iron Company: The area had once housed an iron-smelting industry. Camp would be on the north, or "Sand Shore" of the lake until 1910, when it would be moved to one of Wawayanda's islands.

Scott had to come up with a budget, staff, equipment and camper recruitment plan. The State Committee hadn't allocated any money for the camp, so Charles Kilborne personally financed the first year's venture by writing out a check for $600.

To satisfy campers who had attended Camp Dudley with New York boys for years, the New Jersey Committee opted to run two camps in 1901 – one in July at Wawayanda, and the other in August at Dudley (though they called it Camp Champlain). Following Camp

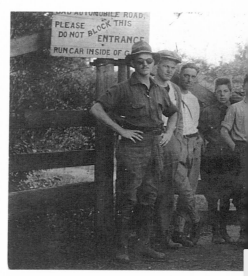

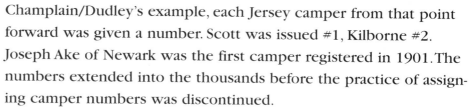

Champlain/Dudley's example, each Jersey camper from that point forward was given a number. Scott was issued #1, Kilborne #2. Joseph Ake of Newark was the first camper registered in 1901. The numbers extended into the thousands before the practice of assigning camper numbers was discontinued.

Dr. Frank North, a teacher at Newark Academy and later Principal at East Side High School in Paterson, N.J., had worked at Camp Dudley for several summers, and served as C. R. Scott's associate during 1901, when energies and attentions were split between two locations. North compiled the camp booklet for 1901, which listed the camp fee of $5 per week at Wawayanda ($5.50 at Champlain), plus reduced round trip train fare of $2 from New York City to Glenwood Glens ($8 to Westport).

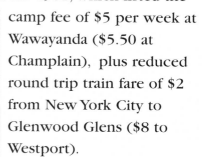

The booklet described the beauties of Wawayanda Lake, noted that "tramping parties" would be scheduled to the "mountains of Sussex County, N.J. and Orange County, N.Y.," and anticipated a "great day in camp" for the Fourth of July, though campers were cautioned not to pack fireworks in with their baggage. At Champlain, excursions to Fort Ticonderoga, Ausable Chasm, and Montreal were slated.

About 75 boys attended each session of camp that year. At Wawayanda, "headquarters" was a 20-by-40-foot canvas tent donated by the Montclair YMCA which had previously used it as a focal point for a fundraising campaign for its new building. The tent became known as the White Elephant at camp, where gusty winds occasionally tore it free from its moorings and across the 1300-foot plateau. Camp Doctor G. Rae Lewis was called upon on more than one occasion to employ waxed twine and stout needles to sew up the big tent's rips and tears.

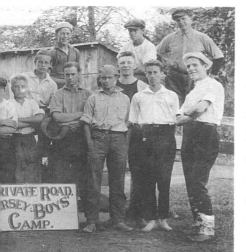

Boys were housed in 16 smaller tents, eight or ten boys per tent, under the supervision of "assistant leaders." These were usually older male volunteers who saw the time at camp as a purposeful vacation. "When you live, eat and sleep with a boy in the open, free life of camp for a month or so, you see sides of his nature which are seldom seen at other times," explained George Hageman, who served as treasurer, counselor and organist at Wawayanda for ten years.

"The cost for board, use of boats and all else pertaining to the Camp is $5.00 per week."

Still, it took some convincing for parents to release their sons to spend the better part of a summer with strangers at camp where the possibility of drowning, illness, broken bones, poison ivy and homesickness were just a few of their worries. A paper prepared by Mrs. Henry Davis for a parents' conference in Ridgewood, N.J. attempted to allay those fears by describing a visit to Wawayanda:

"We were very much impressed with a picture of perhaps 50 boys standing on the edge of the lake with their faces turned upward to the top of the bluff, watching Mr. Scott and waiting for him to blow a whistle as a signal for them to go in the water. When the whistle blew, we could think only of a lot of frightened ducks, diving for safety. It was really a sight worth seeing, bringing out particularly the wonderful command of the director and his perfect control of the boys."

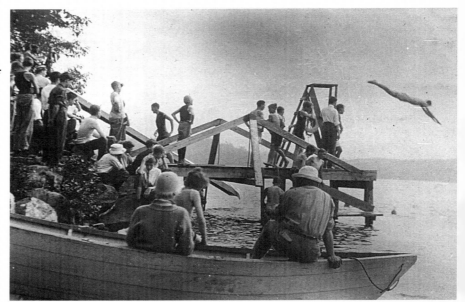

Hearty singing of an appropriate blessing before each meal accompanied by a portable organ; boys "enjoying every mouthful out of agate ware, far more than from fine china at home;" a spirited marshmallow roast around the campfire; and a view of "seven boys wrapped in their blankets, being soothed to sleep by an interesting and instructive story from their leader," concluded Mrs. Davis' description.

Scott's own wife would prove to be the best testimonial for the virtues of summer camping. In 1903, Director Scott married Jean

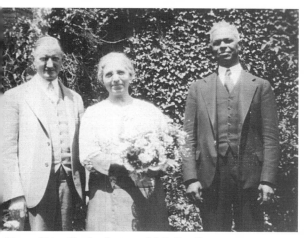

Mr. and Mrs. Charles Scott and R.P. Hamlin

"When camping with children, an oil burner is essential for warming the tent on damp days, or when giving the baby his morning bath. For ironing, an old fashioned charcoal iron is indispensable."

Jean Paterson Scott, "Camp Mother" at Old Wawayanda

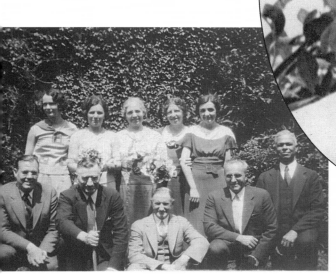

cotts farewell party June 13, 1934
op - Mrs. Froelich, Miss Heiles, Mrs. Scott, Miss Earle, Miss
chneider
ottom - John A. Ledlie, Urban Williams, Charles Scott, E.W. Barnes,
P. Hamlin

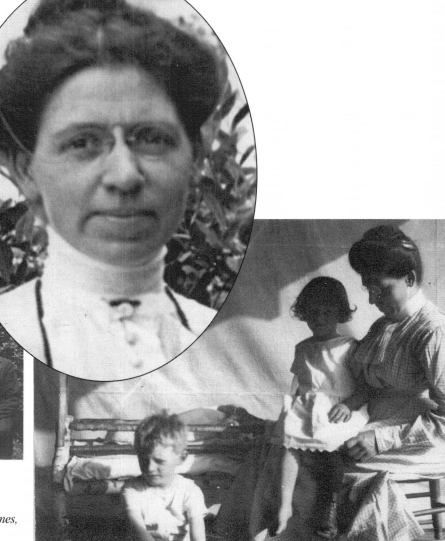

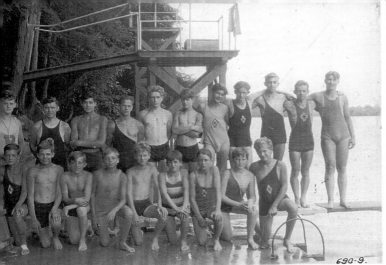

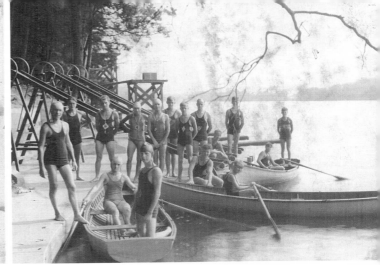

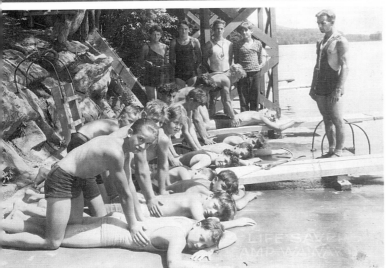

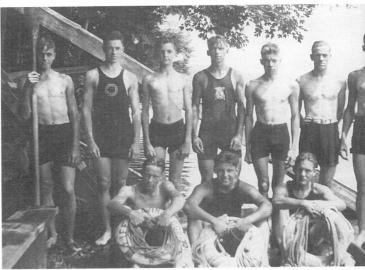

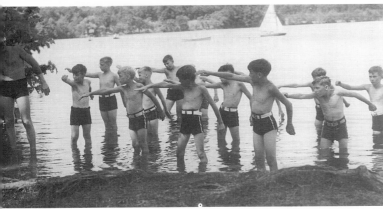

"Every boy a swimmer, every swimmer a lifesaver."

Official slogan of the Lifesaving Corps

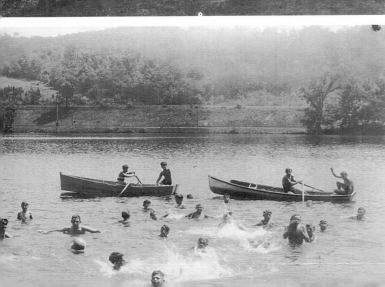

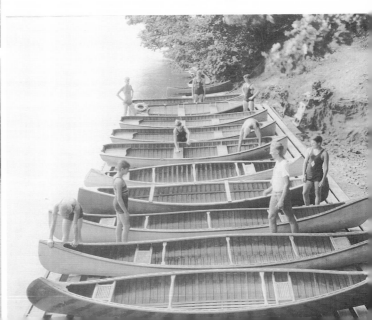

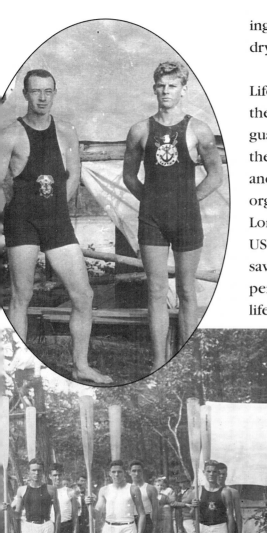

ing boys, among them a jeweler's apprentice, grocery store clerk, laundry boy and an electrician.

Swimming instruction, and a course offered by the U. S. Volunteer Lifesaving Corps, were provided at camp. The USVLSC was formed at the turn of the century by a group of men who served as unpaid lifeguards at Battery Park in New York City. C. R. Scott had approached the group in 1905 about offering instruction in lifesaving techniques and water and boat safety to Wawayanda campers, and then helped organize a systematic program of teaching and testing. W. E. Longfellow, Wawayanda's waterfront director and a member of USVLSC, enlisted Wawayanda to help him with demonstrations of lifesaving methods around the region. Longfellow ultimately helped persuade the Red Cross to develop what would become a national lifesaving and water safety program, and years later hailed Wawayanda as one of the "laboratories" in which this Red Cross staple was developed.

Wawayanda contributed as well to the development of the fledgling Boy Scouts of America soon after the movement spread across the Atlantic from its home in England. Youth workers like C. R. Scott and Frank Gray of the Montclair, N.J. Board of Education, wanted to encourage the values and goals of the Boy Scouts and

ructors McNair & Hagan and a lifesaving drill

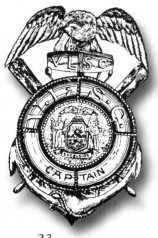

Scout camping, and so participated in the first annual meeting of the National Council of Boy Scouts of America in February, 1911. President William Howard Taft, honorary president of the organization, received the council in the East Room of the White House. That summer, Scott organized a special training program for Boy Scout leaders which was conducted across Lake Wawayanda from the YMCA camp. The Y's State Executive Committee supervised the week-long session, which trained leaders in knot tying, boat management, tracking, signaling and "overnight bivouacking." Participants paid a $2 fee and were advised to bring their own teepee, and leave the tobacco at home.

The Wawayanda camp program also included classes in first aid, signaling and knot tying. There were Field Day contests, skits, and lessons in reading the stars. Photography, with "daylight development and printing," was added by 1909. In all activities, related C. R. Scott, four things were emphasized: Order, cleanliness, respect and service to others.

In 1910, growing attendance spurred the development of a new tent site on an island provided by owner Nelson Graves. Campers slept and held evening services on what became known as "Chapel Island," which was connected by a rope-tow ferry to the mainland where activities and meals were provided. The director's tent, camp office and store were located on the southern point of the island.

The flat-bottomed ferry measured 8x20 feet. Designed by Raymond White, it could only be operated by those riding in it, who pulled on a rope stretched across the water to haul the little craft to the opposite shore. The ferry also served as a floating choir loft for hymn sings.

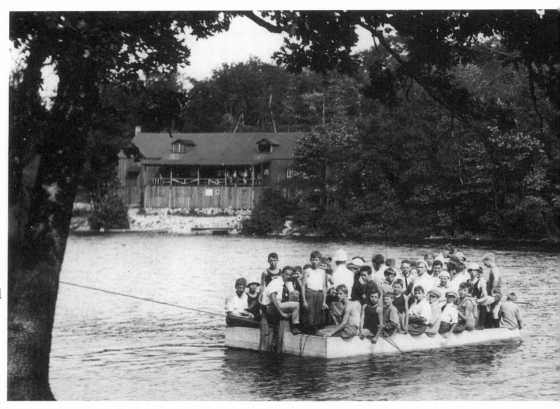

1910 -The famous "Cable Ferry" connected the mainland to "the island". It was built to hold 45 and once ran with 75 aboard! Official record for the crossing - 37 seconds!

The first trip to camp by an automobile was made by a Bernardsville group in 1911. By 1915, the Y's Women's Auxiliary had collected enough money to purchase a camp car, a Model T. The first drivers were Donald Richmond and Mervin Hall.

Holding sway over the camp kitchen for the first several years was A. Y. Allen of Trenton, who had served as one of the cooks at The Breakers Resort at Palm Beach, Florida. Local produce and dairy products were utilized, and in 1912, the camp purchased several lambs which were slaughtered for food. Some campers learned the craft of

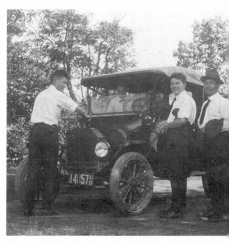

Some New Jersey Y.M.C.A. Boys
:: WHO HAVE ADVANCED ::
Into the Service of Their Country

Y.M.C.A.

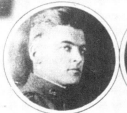

LIEUT. OSCAR B. LEWIS
Cranford
U. S. Aviation Service

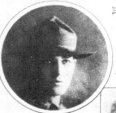

LIEUT. DAVID ACKERMAN
Passaic
312th Field Artillery

THOMAS D. OS-
BOURNE, Cranford
U. S. S. Solace

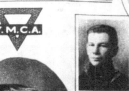

STATE SECRETARY CHARLES R. SCOTT
Whose Silver Anniversary as Y. M. C. A. Secretary Was Celebrated at Banquet Here on Thursday

AUSTIN H. WHE-
DON, Ridgewood
U. S. S. Conyngham

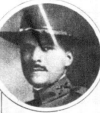

LIEUT. J. NORMAN DOWNER
Orange
Co. D, 62d Inf

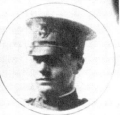

LIEUT. JOHN K. MERRILL
Plainfield
Base Hospital, A. E. F

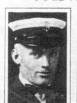

TICE C. LOBBREGT
Paterson
Naval Reserve

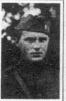

LIEUT. CLARENCE D
BAILEY, Summit
Instructor, A. E. F

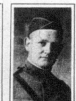

LIEUT. JOHN E.
THROCKMORTON, Co. E,
115th Inf., 29th Division
A. E. F

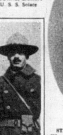

MAJOR WALDEN H. McNAIR
Camp Lee, Va.

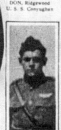

LIEUT. H. HALLOCK BROWN
Aviation, A. E. F

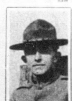

LIEUT. ROBERT B. HILL
Orange
Killed April 29, 1918

LIEUT. J. C. NEFF
High Bridge
308th Machine Gun Co

HOWARD S. LYON
Perth Amboy
Naval Reserve

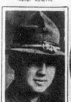

JOHN M. HAMPTON
Cranford
42th Motor Truck Co.

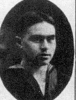

WILLIAM BROWER
West Orange
U. S. S. Kemah

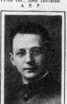

CHARLES F. DAHLGREN
East Orange
Infantry, A. E. F

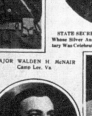

RAYMOND MANLEY
Plainfield
Ambulance Driver

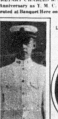

FREDERICK CLAY
Plainfield
U. S. Navy

JOHN D. MOORE
Haddonfield
A. E. F

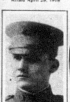

E. H. ELLIS
Paterson
U. S. Aviation Service

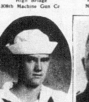

RONALD HELPS
Montclair
Naval Reserves

WILLIAM P. COUSE
Asbury Park
Battery F, 112th H. F. A.

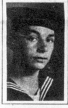

FLOYD STAGE
Wawayanda
U. S. S. New Jersey

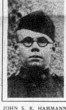

JOHN S. K. HAMMANN
Plainfield
Battery D, 105th F A

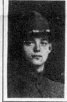

SERGT. T W HERMAN
Plainfield
U S Hospital Corps

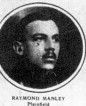

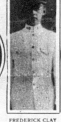

HERBERT KNIGHT
Montclair
U. S. S. C. 235

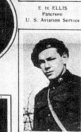

MILES A. SUAREZ
Orange
Killed on Marne, July 15

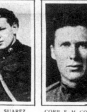

CORP E. H. COUSINS
Belleville
Battery E, 112th H F A

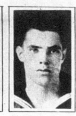

CHARLES A. BIRD JR.
Elizabeth
U. S. Navy

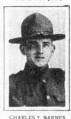

CHARLES Y. BARNES
Madison
Wounded April 12, 1918

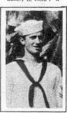

ROBERT K. KEE
Orange
U. S. Navy

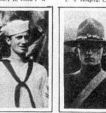

HAROLD W. TOMLIN-
SON, Plainfield
Medical Corps, A. E. F.

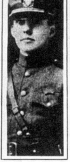

ENSIGN J. CLEMENT
BOYD, Montclair
U. S. Naval Air Service

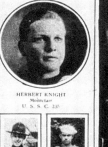

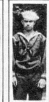

LIEUT JAMES VALEN-
TINE JR. Glen Ridge
Royal Air Force

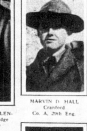

MARVIN D. HALL
Cranford
Co. A, 29th Eng.

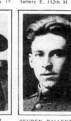

REUBEN BALLENTINE
Summit
Infantry, A. E. F

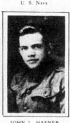

JOHN L. HAFNER
Plainfield
Co. B, 104th Eng

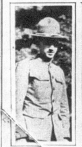

SERGT. T. WALDEN
FOUNTAIN, Elizabeth
Co. C, 311th

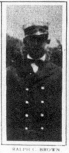

RALPH C. BROWN
Bernardsville
Naval Reserves

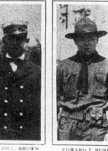

EDWARD T. BURR
Cranford
4th Field Artillery

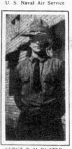

SERGT. B. H. BUTTER-
FIELD, Jersey City
Co. A, 312th Inf

SERGT ARTHUR
C. BIRD, Passaic
303d Engineers

PAUL F. FEN-
TON, Metuchen
U. S. Navy

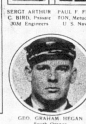

GEO. GRAHAM HEGAN
South Orange
U. S. N. R. F.

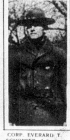

CORP. EVERARD T.
SCHOPPER, Arlington
Co. C, 302d Eng.

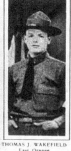

THOMAS J. WAKEFIELD
East Orange
Croix de Guerre, June, 1918

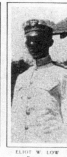

ELIOT W. LOW
Paterson
U. S. S. Michigan

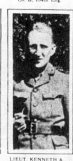

LIEUT. KENNETH A.
BAILEY, Glen Ridge
102d Field Artillery

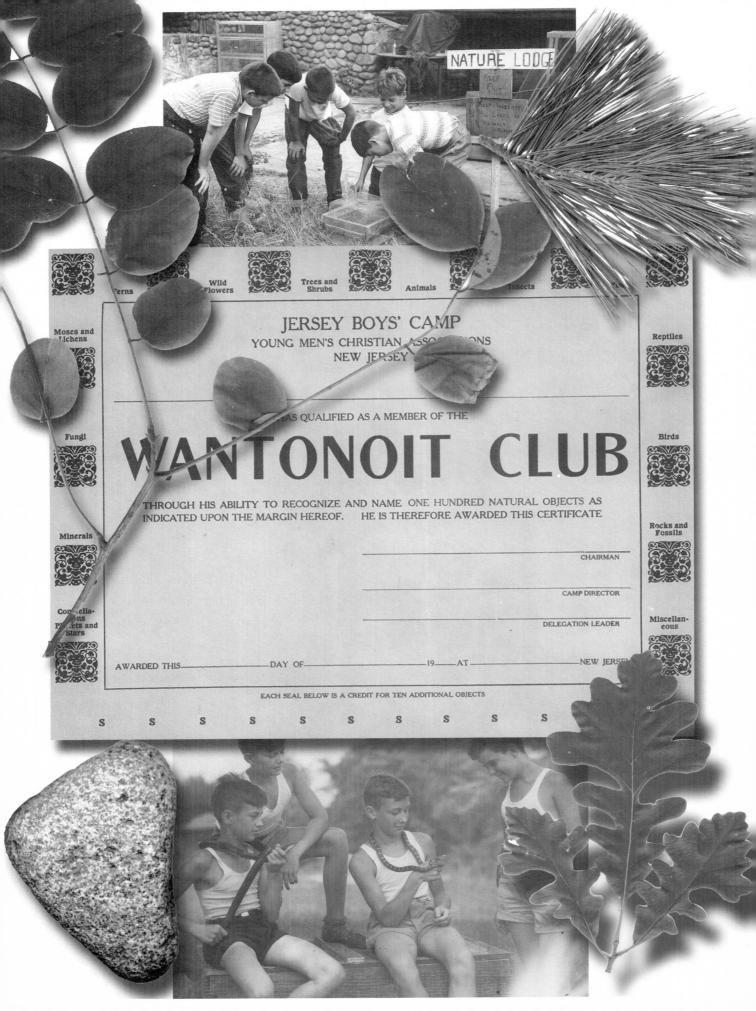

Ferns | Wild Flowers | Trees and Shrubs | Animals | Insects

Mosses and Lichens

Fungi

Minerals

Constellations Planets and Stars

JERSEY BOYS' CAMP
YOUNG MEN'S CHRISTIAN ASSOCIATIONS
NEW JERSEY

HAS QUALIFIED AS A MEMBER OF THE

WANTONOIT CLUB

THROUGH HIS ABILITY TO RECOGNIZE AND NAME ONE HUNDRED NATURAL OBJECTS AS
INDICATED UPON THE MARGIN HEREOF.   HE IS THEREFORE AWARDED THIS CERTIFICATE

CHAIRMAN

CAMP DIRECTOR

DELEGATION LEADER

AWARDED THIS_____DAY OF_____19___AT_____NEW JERSEY

EACH SEAL BELOW IS A CREDIT FOR TEN ADDITIONAL OBJECTS

S   S   S   S   S   S   S   S   S

Reptiles

Birds

Rocks and Fossils

Miscellaneous

NATURE LODGE

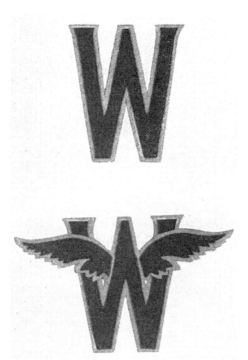

tanning as they cured the lamb pelts for rugs.

Jean Scott's father, Robert Paterson, was a familiar figure around camp, using his mechanic's skills to repair equipment, buildings, boats and plumbing, and teaching tool use to campers. Known as "Old Faithful," he was remembered for his sense of humor, his sound advice, and for his heartfelt renditions of songs from his native Scotland.

A camp newsletter, *The Wawayanda Whirlwind*, kept campers and leaders in touch with goings-on from the very beginning. Walter H. Wones, who later succeeded C. R. Scott as Boys Work Secretary of the Newark Y, wrote the first edition by hand in 1901. The following season, the newsletter was duplicated on the "hextograph," which was succeeded by the Edison mimeograph. Then, the nearby *Warwick Dispatch* devoted a section of the weekly newspaper to camp activities and gave each camper a complimentary copy. *The Whirlwind* was published for decades to come.

By 1917, Camp Wawayanda included a two-room, open-sided "school house" overlooking the lake where summer school classes in mathematics and other subjects were conducted. A cabin, funded by the Ridgewood YMCA Women's Auxiliary, served as the office, and a boat house doubled as a store near the ferry landing. There was also a hospital tent. A Japanese cook was the chef, and more than 50 leaders, including clergymen, teachers, chemists, draftsmen, dentists, real estate agents and bankers, served as unpaid counselors.

On Saturday nights, special guests presented stereopticon lectures. Prof. W. H. Browne of Colby College organized the Wantonoit Club, which awarded certificates to campers who could recognize and name 100 or more objects from nature. An honor emblem, the Wawayanda W, was given to boys who secured 100 points from a list of physical, social, educational and craft activities. Moral achievements, such as "helping the other fellow," and "faithful participation in Bible study and Sunday services," also earned points toward the W, and a follow-up award known as "Wings."

The cost for boys 12 to 18 was $8 per week, and four two-week sessions were offered. By then more than 2,500 Jersey boys had attended camp, and a campaign was underway to purchase a perma-

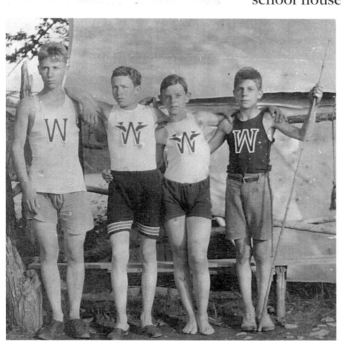

The Wawayanda "W" which is the honor emblem of the Camp, will be awarded to the campers who have secured 100 points in the following tests: Physical, Social, Educational, Moral, Camp and Woodcraft. Boys who failed last season are credited with points which hold good this season.

nent camp site, since the existing property had been purchased by the N. J. Zinc Company.

Camp continued through 1918, when the rumblings of World War I could be felt even on the tranquil shores of Lake Wawayanda. "Feeding hungry campers that season was difficult, for cooks were urgently required by the Army," related Hugh Scott. "During the ten-week camping period, 18 different cooks were employed to cook for Wawayanda campers. Some served only a few days before being drafted for military service." Hugh's mother, Jean Scott, was pressed into service cooking for camp for ten straight days, "developing recipes by equating all ingredients to her familiar family-of-five standards," her son recalled.

Father C. R. Scott received countless letters from and about former campers who had been wounded or killed in the fighting in Europe. The letters, he later wrote, "made a deep impression on our family and campers for we were knit together in camp as one big family." On one occasion, a Passaic Army captain brought a sleeping bag and several personal articles of former camper and war casualty William Marselis, Jr. to a Saturday night

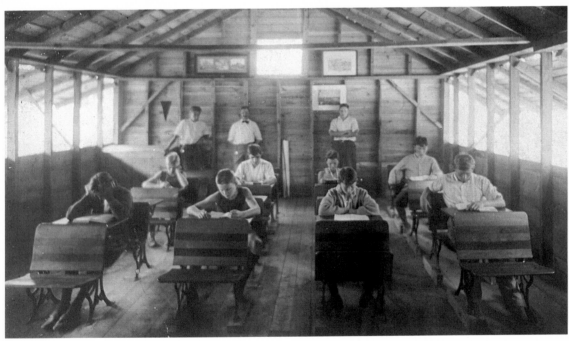

Open-sided schoolhouse where boys could brush up on fundamentals.

Council Ring. Among the items displayed in the dim light of the dying fire was Marselis' Bible, which was used for years afterwards in camp and at conferences.

Change was in the wind for Wawayanda as the world set its sights on peace in 1919.

A chance encounter on a street corner in Newton, N.J. led to the purchase of Camp Wawayanda's new home in 1919.

That January, Charles R. Scott and Albert Kennelly, who with other State Committeemen had been searching for a new home for the camp since 1917, took the train to Newton to visit a potential site at Sucker Pond in Sussex County. When they arrived, they found that heavy snows, followed by a thaw, had made the roads to the site impassable. A passerby overheard the men discussing the situation, and interjected that a nearby estate with a lovely pond was on the market if they were interested. He directed them to the real estate agent handling the property, and an immediate inspection of the 330-acre Slater Estate was arranged.

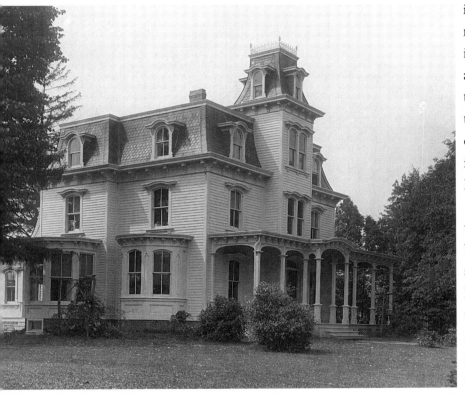

Purchased in 1919, the 10 bedroom house became "Ayer Hall" and was transformed into an inn which accommodated guests, Y meetings and conferences.

Frank Slater gave the Y visitors a tour of the site, which included a 10-bedroom main house, a tenant house and cottage, a large barn, a carriage house and boathouses on the estate's two lakes. The asking price was $50,000, but, related Scott, since "the Slater family was especially pleased that their old home and lakes would be considered for such work as the Young Men's Christian Association," it came down to $40,000 by the end of that first visit. Following a second visit in the company of Asbury banker William Couse, chairman of the New Jersey State Executive Committee, the price was further reduced to $30,000. The State Committee approved the purchase, and the sale was finalized March 21, with about $12,000 of the needed funds already in hand from generous benefactors, including Mr. Couse, who contributed the first $600, Mr. and Mrs. Archibald Bull, Elizabeth and Samuel Hird, State Committee Chairman F. Wayland Ayer, Austin Colgate, James McCutheon and S. J. McCawley. Charles Kilborne, who had so readily launched the first camp with a personal donation, once again dug into his own pockets and encouraged others to do so.

The purchase set into motion a busy spring of arranging facilities and equipment, engaging leaders, enrolling campers, raising additional funds and outlining a plan for the new facility. Less than three months after the New Jersey YMCA took title to the Slater Estate, Camp Wawayanda completed the move to its new location on June 13. The hand-pulled ferry at the old camp was pressed into service carrying building parts and furnishings from the island, across Lake Wawayanda to the mainland and on to the new camp more than 20 miles away.

New Wawayanda, 60 miles from New York City and Trenton, 100 miles from Camden, and only a mile-and-a-half from the Andover station of the Delaware, Lackawanna and Western Railroad, was indeed a perfect place for a summer camp. The site included 90 acres of farmland, 100 acres of woodland, and two lakes. The 117-acre Long Pond, at 110 to 135 feet deep perhaps the deepest in New Jersey, had a natural sand bar, ideal for a bathing beach. The lake abounded with bass, perch and rainbow trout. The smaller Hewitt Pond was connected to the larger water body by a quarter-mile-long stream. A large field overlooking the lake provided plenty of space for games and recreation.

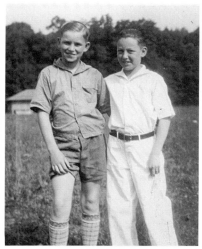
Campers George Nielsen & Weston Lucas

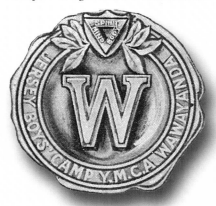

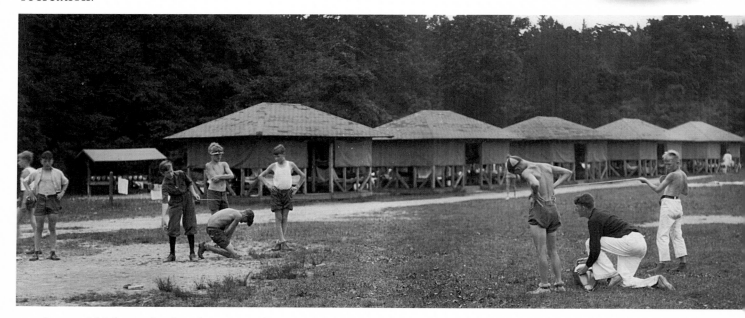

Some 100 boys had to be turned away from New Wawayanda during its first summer of operation for lack of accommodations on "tent row." Improvements were made and facilities added as the State Committee worked to collect the $100,000 needed to repair and

Main Lodge

maintain existing buildings, pay off the purchase debt and create a camp endowment fund.

The need for a lodge, with dining hall and assembly room to hold 200 people, was apparent from the start, and the 1919 campers almost immediately launched a campaign to raise the money to build one. The lodge, equipped with a handsome stone fireplace and an old locomotive bell that called campers to mess or worship, was finished a year later, dedicated to the 486 former Wawayanda campers who had served in World War I, and in memory of 16 who did not return.

The stately Slater mansion was transformed into an "inn" called "Ayer Hall" that accommodated guests, Y meetings and conferences. "This gives the enjoyment of camp with all the conveniences of home," said a 1922 camp booklet. In 1924, a gift from Samuel Hird, a New Jersey woolen manufacturer and YMCA supporter who had contributed toward YMCA buildings in Passiac and Garfield, N.J., made possible the building of a boathouse and a concrete swimming dock at Wawayanda. The dock was equipped with diving boards and slides and supervised by certified Red Cross life savers.

In 1926, an outdoor chapel in a serene pine grove was erected as a tribute to Charles Kilborne. A quarter-century earlier, Kilborne had named Charles R. Scott as the first New Jersey Boys Work

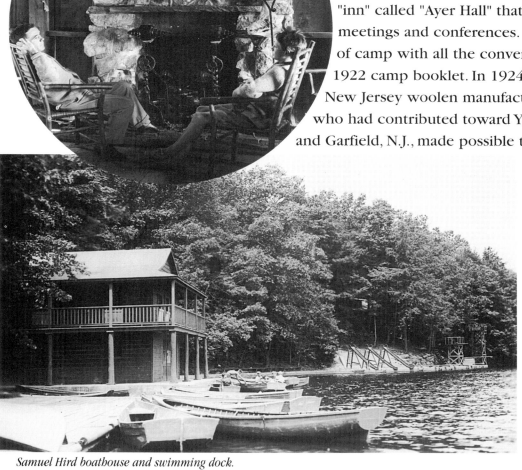

Samuel Hird boathouse and swimming dock.

Secretary, setting in motion the development of Camp Wawayanda at its original location.

Scott had retired as Wawayanda camp director in 1921. A 10-month, 24-country world tour to promote the YMCA and the development of missionary, recreational and health programs for youth in Asia, Europe and Africa had convinced him that his energies should have a broader focus. So the man who founded Wawayanda turned over the camp reins to William MacCormick, the first of five camp directors to hold the post over the next nine years.

Scott remained State Boys Work Secretary until his retirement from the Y in 1934. In addition to his achievements with Camp Wawayanda, he was first president of the Camp Directors Association of America. At the time of his retirement, it was called the American Camping Association and had 5,400 member camps serving more than five million campers in the U.S. In 1930, Scott gained considerable fame when he compiled a booklet titled "Larry, Thoughts of Youth" made up of inspirational letters, poems and essays written by former Wawayanda camper Larimore Foster, who was killed in a horseback riding accident in 1925. "Larry" was published by the Y's Association Press, and more than a million copies were sold to YMCAs and other organizations and individuals around the world. Scott conducted an exhaustive nationwide speaking tour on behalf of Larry and the fine attributes he represented.

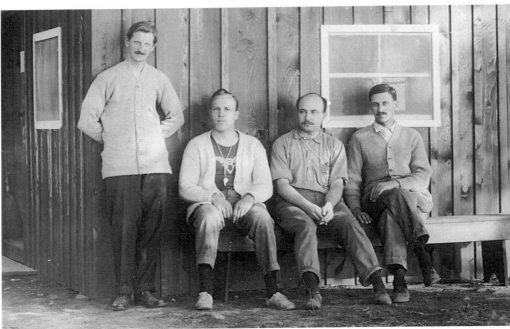

C.R. Scott, standing, and the headquarters crew.

Even after retirement in 1934, Scott maintained an active life, never losing his great affection for Wawayanda and the boys he had seen mature there. Camp sights and sounds colored his memories into old age. In 1948, he remembered "laughter, splashing water, a crackling fire, the rattle of dishes, running feet, the crack of a bat against a ball, bugle calls . . . chopping wood, cleaning lanterns, peeling potatoes and freezing ice cream, overnight parties to Haunted Cabin Point, dark dramatics and mock trials, airplane and model boat

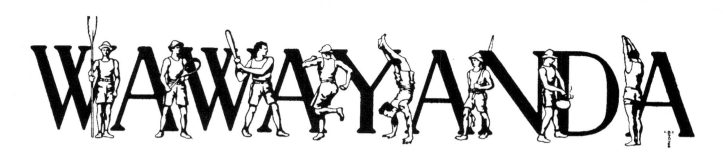

building, chapel programs and campfires of pure delight. . ."

Such activities continued, of course, after Scott's departure from the daily Wawayanda scene. In 1926, 590 campers signed up for one- or two-week sessions running from June 23 to Sept. 1. New Jersey boys between 12 and 18 could attend for $12 per week

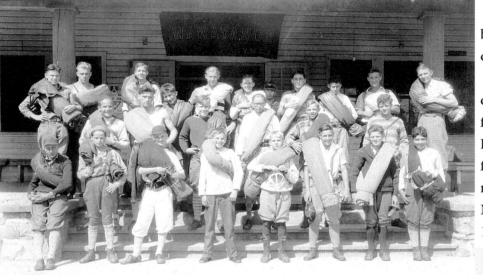

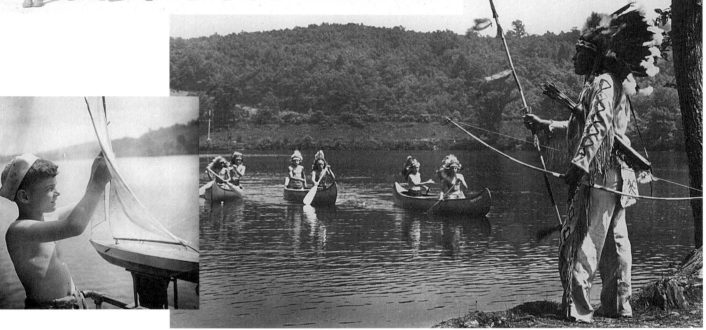

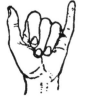

The Wawayanda Salute

plus a $3 registration fee. (The youngest allowable age was subsequently lowered to nine.) "No rebates can be granted to those who arrive late, are dismissed, or withdraw except in case of sickness – homesickness not included," explained the 1927 brochure.

"Everything a boy likes to do is found at Wawayanda," proclaimed a 1933 brochure, which listed track events, canoeing, hiking, Indian

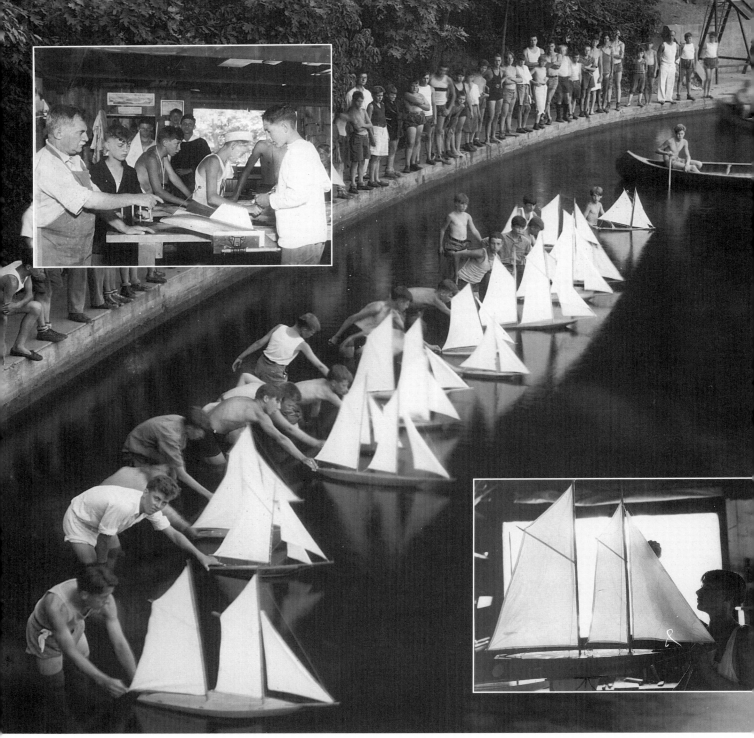

lore, camp cooking, even harmonica playing among them. There
were ball fields, horseshoe pits, basketball courts, archery and shoot-
ing ranges, and several very busy tennis courts. There was an "opera
house" where singing, dramatics and an "orchestra" held sway. Music
"taken from the air" was also heard on a camp radio set built in
1922. On February 19 that year, C. R. Scott delivered his "Boys of the
World" address over the fledgling airwaves of Newark radio station
WJZ, gaining national recognition for originating a wireless broadcast

*Captain Saunders' Craft Shop going full
steam in the production of model boats -
and the results.*

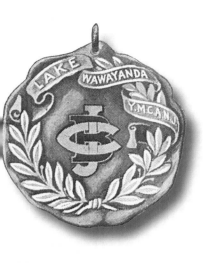

relayed over a 2,000 mile radius.

Woodcraft, belt making and "Apache bead work" were favorites in the campcraft arena. According to 1930s camper and staff member Ed Ewen, a former ship captain taught model boat building and a Native American known as Chief White Bear taught Indian lore. Campers over the years made everything from birdhouses to wallets to hot dog forks and andirons hammered into shape over a specially made forge. Camper-built kayaks competed for space on the lake, and hand-made jewelry, including the Wawayanda Special – a bracelet with the head of an Indian upon it – was often lost beneath the waves during swimming and boating outings. Al Chrone, also a camper in the mid-1930s, remembers searching the "Sink Easy," the name given to the shallow area of the waterfront, in an effort to find the lost ring of his Japanese counselor.

Scouting for arrowheads in the camp's farm fields, or fool's gold and garnet crystals in the nearby Andover iron ore mines, were favorite adventures. The mines, originally worked by the British and the Colonial Armies during the Revolution, were last plumbed during World War II and remain a feature of what is now Kittatinny Valley State Park.

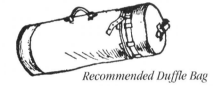

Recommended Duffle Bag

Campers were advised to bring rainwear to camp, along with flannel pajamas, two pairs of heavy blankets, "hard water soap that will float," a bathing suit, athletic shorts and shirts, sewing supplies, a collapsible drinking cup, a Bible and a "cheerful disposition."

Tent houses – partially enclosed canvas-covered living units – accommodated campers. F. W. "Batchy" Holbein, assistant director of

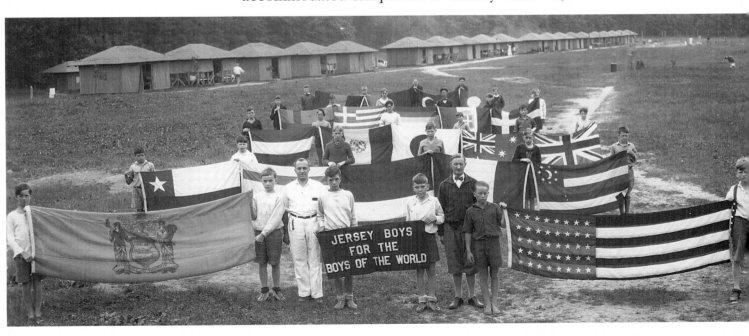

the camp from 1928 to 1949, remembered that when he arrived in 1928, there was a row of 20 tent houses on the west side of campus, while five identical structures, called "Millionaire's Row" located near the lake shore, housed older campers. "Behind each row of tent houses was a road which brought copious dust to the living quarters during hot, dry weather, and masses of mud on rainy days," Holbein recalled.

The linear tent arrangement gave way in the early 1930s to the village concept, proposed and promoted to the wider YMCA audience by John A. Ledlie, Wawayanda's director from 1930 to 1945. Clusters of tents, later cabins, were grouped four or six to a "village," allowing different age groups to live together in a sort of mini-camp which included toilet facilities and a meeting lodge. This "decentralization" model was borrowed from the National Park Service, which in 1930 constructed several widely scattered "Recreation Demonstration Projects," each with four to six cabins, wash house, and lodge. The YMCA was influenced by this experiment, and Wawayanda was the first of the Y camps to implement the village model in 1934. Many others soon followed.

Similarly, new concepts in educational theory were

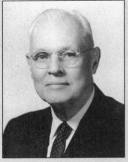

John A. Ledlie, 1898-1975

"John always does things right." An associate once made that simple assertion about John A. Ledlie, who did indeed enjoy an extraordinarily successful career as a YMCA youth director, program developer, policy maker and author. He spent nearly 50 years with the Y, 15 of them as Director of Camp Wawayanda, where he instituted several innovations, including the arrangement of tents into age-based "villages." As Youth and Camping Secretary for the National Council of YMCAs from 1944 to 1963, Ledlie developed national standards for camp health, safety and sanitation, counselor training, and administration. A scholar and educator, he authored more than two dozen books, articles and monographs on topics ranging from camp design to wilderness skills to youth and family issues. He was widely recognized as an authority on camp management and his ideas – many of them formulated at Camp Wawayanda – were adopted by camps nationwide.

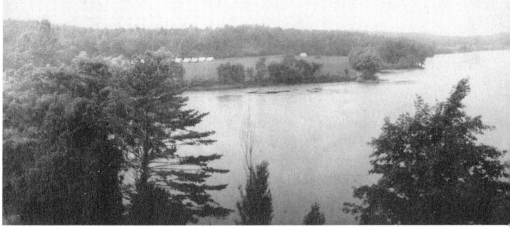

reflected in the shift from military-styled camp lay-out, and regimented programming and scheduling, to a more democratic system of camp administration, physical arrangement and leadership training. *Camping and Character*, a 1929 book by Hedley Dimock and Charles Hendry published by the YMCA, explained how educational principles could be applied to camp activities so that camps could

*"Dear old Wawayanda,
How I love thy shores,
With their fringing forests
Where the wild bird soars.*

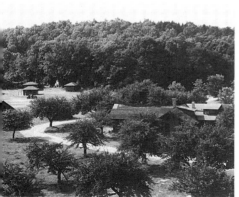

The results of John Ledlie's village concept.

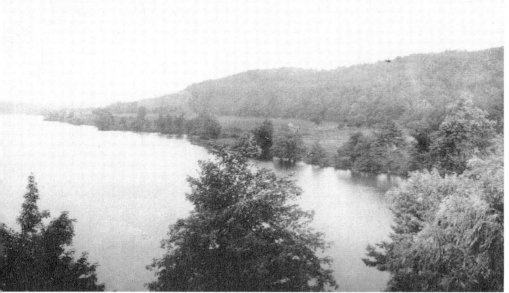

Island dotted picture, full of charm for me, Ever glad the moment I may turn to thee."

One of several songs written in tribute to Lake Wawayanda.

stimulate intellect, imagination and personality growth, beyond serving as healthful recreational outlets and religious training centers. Organizing tents and cabins in smaller groups, with a senior counselor, or "village chief" at the top of the totem pole, allowed more age-specific programming, a tighter camp "family," and the institution of democratic "councils" at which village residents could learn to govern themselves, share responsibility and resolve differences, thus building better citizens.

Wawayanda embraced this model and under Ledlie's able leadership, rearranged the camp's lay-out and its operational structure. Tents were clustered in six age-related villages, named Outpost, Totem, Forest, Lenape, Hemlock and Pioneer. Programs were graded to the interests and needs of the residents. Campers selected officers like the Sachem and the Scribe. They were involved more fully in making decisions affecting their tents or cabins and the village at large. And counselors participated in planning their own training experiences.

Those counselors took their cue from the *Camp Counselor's Manual*, written in 1937 by Ledlie and Assistant Camp Director Holbein. The manual was one of more than a dozen books on camp administration, programming and standards written or edited by Ledlie, who went on to become Youth Program and Camping Secretary for the National Council of YMCAs until his 1963 retirement from the Y. The book listed several essential qualifications of a good camp counselor. These included a genuine liking of boys, a love of the outdoors, attention to health and safety issues, proficiency in some skill and the ability to teach it, and some understanding of child development. A counselor should also have "a personal and social philosophy based on the teachings of Jesus," the manual advised.

Prospective counselors were given a list of reference books such as "How to Make Recurve Bows and Matched Arrows," "Fun with Skits, Stunts and Stories," "Good Times Around the Campfire" and

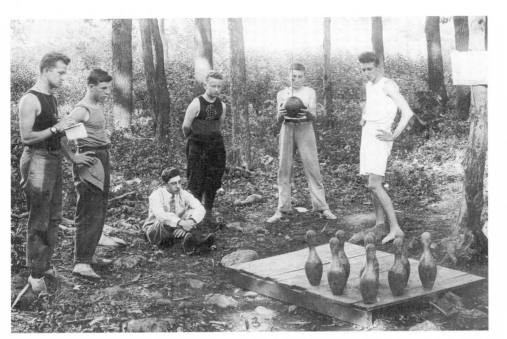

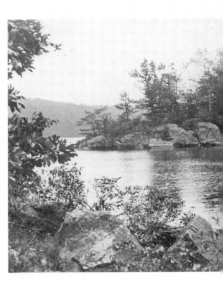

CAMP ACTIVITIES

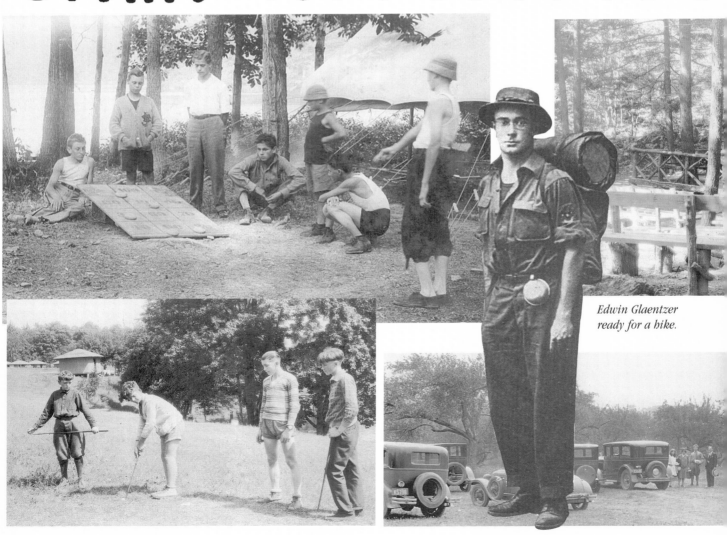

*Edwin Glaentzer
ready for a hike.*

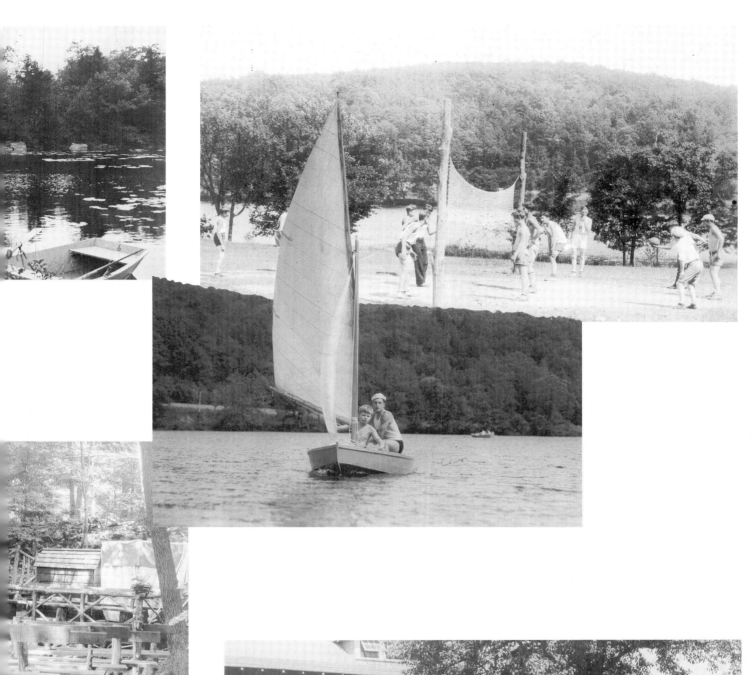

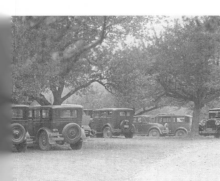

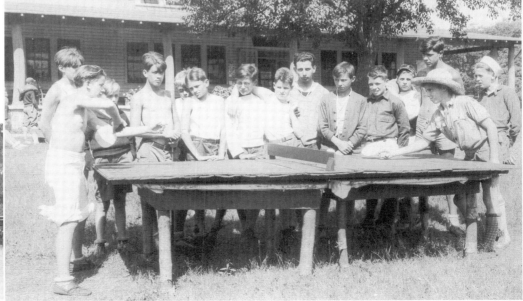

"100 Devotions for Boys and Girls." The manual included a self-exam in which the counselor rated his emotional age ("Are you hotheaded . . . given to gossip . . . showing personal predjudice . . . unable to plan ahead . . .?") It described small group games like Blindfold Boxing, Badger Pull and Are You There, Waddie? It also offered advice on using daily camp experiences to initiate evening scripture readings or spiritual discussions.

Allowing their charges to organize and implement programs and activities did not come easily to some counselors. A few, wrote Frank Essig, chief of the older boys' village at Wawayanda in 1940, "still had a hangover of benevolent paternalism in dealing with their boys."

But the democratic notion prevailed. Soon, the boys had revamped an honors program they felt sometimes rewarded with the coveted "W" boys who had not worked hard enough for it; revived the Wakon-Kitchewah, a leadership society for 15-and 16-year-olds which also edited the thrice-weekly *Wawayanda Wasp* newspaper; and formed a junior chapter of the leadership organization, called the Questapa Society (Fellowship of Little Chiefs), which took on as its first project construction of a log lean-to in an isolated part of camp where meetings and overnights were held.

Through the years, camp facilities and infrastructure were improved. In 1932, a new infirmary was added with financial assistance from the YMCA's Women's Auxiliary. The Auxiliary also furnished Ayer Hall as a guest house, supplied libraries in several village lodges, replaced dining and kitchen ware, and purchased a new public address system. New sanitation and electrical systems were installed. A home was built on campus for the camp director and his family.

In 1946, a new $10,000 kitchen, paid for with donations, was added with an enlarged bakery, gas stoves to replace the old coal-fired one, and a 50-gallon steam kettle for preparing countless potatoes and ears of corn.

Summer school classes continued to be offered at New Wawayanda. They were conducted in the boathouse named Normandie Lodge after it was renovated to include double-decker bunks made from remnants of the French liner Normandie which burned in 1942 while being outfitted as a military transport in New York City.

The war years were seen as an opportunity to promote "resourcefulness in the out-of-doors, responsibility in cooperative living, and ruggedness in physical and mental conditioning," explained

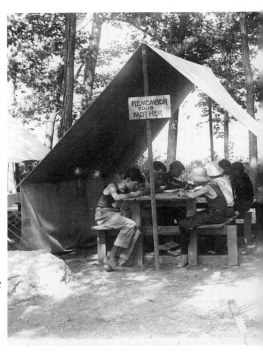

WRITE HOME FREQUENTLY
"In the dear old home they miss you
Miss the sunshine of your face,
Miss your happy careless chatter:
No one else can fill your place.
They are thinking of you often
When in distant paths you roam:
Don't forget to write a letter
To the dear ones left at home."

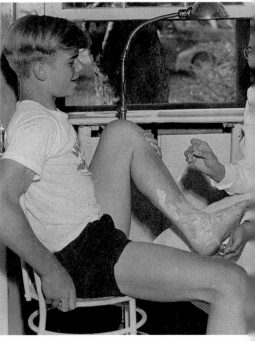

Camper Robert Glen Smith and Nurse Voorees

the 1943 camp brochure. "In the days ahead, boys will be called upon to assume many responsibilities that formerly were carried by adults . . . (and) in a few short years, some of our present day campers will be called upon to help solve the pressing problems in making a peaceful world." The brochure quoted a former Wawayanda camper, then in the service, who declared that his experience at camp helped prepare him for close-quarters living in the Army. The new "democratic training" endorsed by Wawayanda, the brochure added, also gave young people "the ability to think straight, to express one's point of view without rancor (and) to adjust to new persons and situations."

Wawayanda alumni in Europe, the Pacific or in Africa stayed abreast of camp activities through the efforts of Batchy Holbein. The assistant camp director, who was for many years an administrator for Mt. Holly (N.J.) schools compiled the "Wawayanda Service Letter" and distributed it to hundreds of servicemen during the war years; 748 former campers served in all branches of the military, and 28 of them were killed. After the conflict, a new lodge was built in Outpost Village in memory of those who had sacrificed their lives.

Mr. & Mrs. John Ledlie and Batchy Holbein

During World War II Batchy Holbein compiled and distributed hundreds of copies of the "Wawayanda Service Letter" which kept former campers serving in the war in touch with the happenings at Camp Wawayanda. There are many testimonial letters from these soldiers and sailors expressing just how important that connection was to them.

F.W. "Batchy" Holbein

"Friendly, understanding, patient - these are a few of the qualities which are remembered by those who passed through Wawayanda during the years 1928-1949, of Mr. F.W. Holbein, better known as Batchy.

Batchy had that admirable quality of helping everyone to mature without the individual realizing that such maturation was occuring. Wawayanda, through Batchy, grew because of the numerous innovations he helped to institute."

Excerpt from Wawayand Whirlwind 50th Anniversary Issue.

World peace was ever on the mind of an aging Charles R. Scott, who proposed that for the 50th anniversary of Wawayanda's founding in 1951, a Circle of Friendship be constructed at camp made of stones and objects from around the world. He had spent years embedding such items and their histories in concrete blocks at his home in Clifton, N.J., and thought a similar installation would be a nice addition to Wawayanda. The foundation of the circle was laid of native rocks by the side of the lake in a 1948 camp ceremony that involved an American Indian, representatives from Iran, Germany, Japan, Puerto Rico and Venezuela, and other visitors. Also participating were outgoing camp director Alden Eberly and his successor, J. Edward Dodd.

Over the next few years, token rocks and minerals from such sites as the boyhood homes of Jesus in Nazareth, and George Washington in Virginia; from Plymouth Rock; and from Switzerland, Belgium and Norway, were sent in to Scott to be affixed to the Circle of Friendship. Someone contributed a replica of the Rock of Gibraltar, another a piece of petrified wood from Arizona. A rock from Old Wawayanda was placed there, too. But the circle was never completed, and many of the rocks and minerals are believed to have been unknowingly discarded.

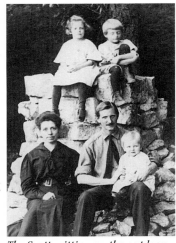

The Scotts sitting on the outdoor pulpit

C. R. Scott's eyesight and hearing faded in his last years, "Mother" Scott became his eyes and ears, helping him correspond with colleagues and former campers. The Scotts marked their 50th wedding anniversary in 1953, and the following summer, Charles R. Scott, 81, died of a heart attack while visiting his beloved Camp Wawayanda. It was the conclusion of a long and productive life in the service of the young people of New Jersey and the world. And it was the end of an era for Camp Wawayanda, now run by the Central Atlantic Area Council of YMCAs, which included Delaware, Maryland, Washington, D.C. and Puerto Rico, as well as New Jersey.

Difficult decisions, and major changes, were just ahead.

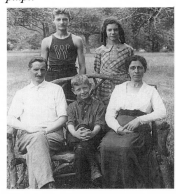

Charles, Bobby and Mother Scott, standing, Hugh and Ruth

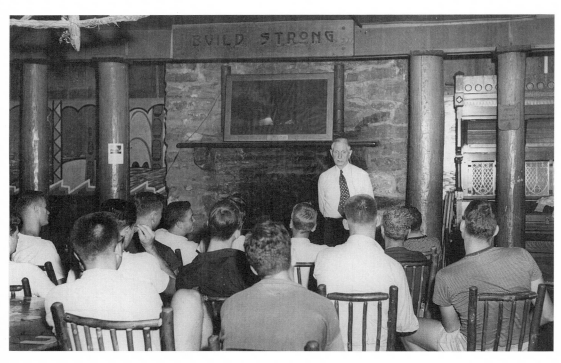

Charles Scott addresses the counselors at Camp Wawayanda just prior to his death.

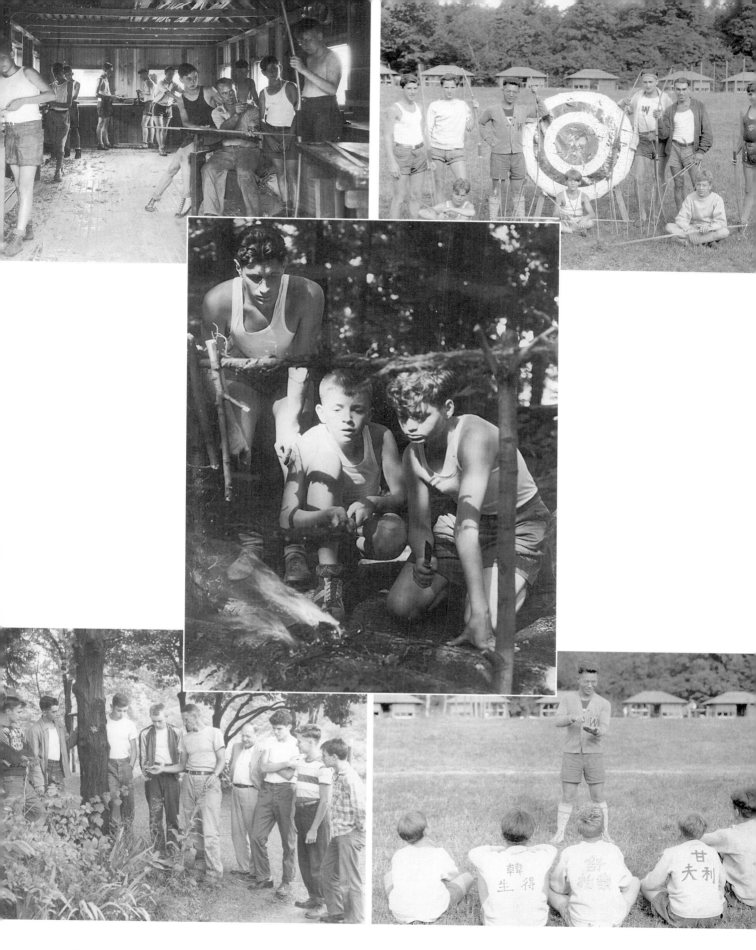

43

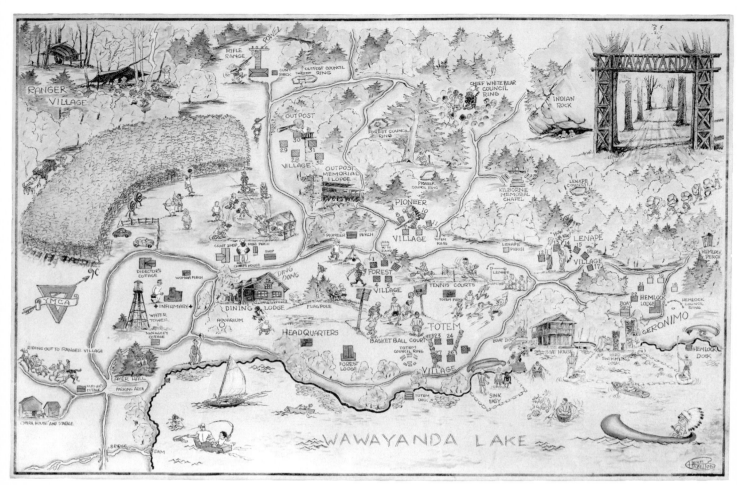

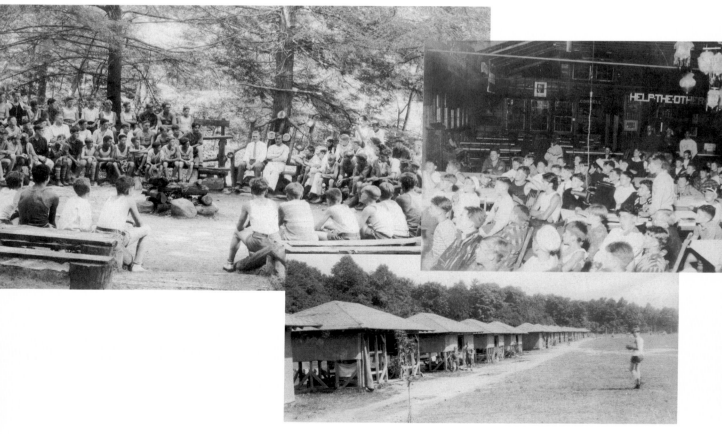

1901 WAWAYANDA — FROST VALLEY 2001

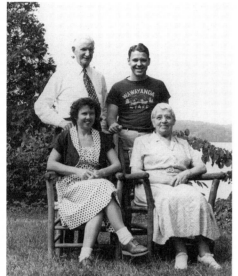

Earl & Bea Armstrong, Camp Directors of Wawayanda, visit with the Scotts.

A s it happened, Charles R. Scott died during Wawayanda's last summer at Andover.

In the mid-1950s, the "community was closing in" on the New Jersey facility. "It was becoming too civilized for a boys' camp," recalled Earl Armstrong, Camping Executive for the Central Atlantic Area Council of YMCAs (CAAC). Armstrong, who had previously worked for YMCAs in South Carolina and Kentucky, served as Director of Wawayanda and another Y camp, Camp Speers in Dingman's Ferry, Pennsylvania, from 1953 to 1956.

"For some time, we have felt the growing community around us, have noted the additional traffic by road and rail, have seen more and more use of our lake by outsiders as we tried to give boys a truly significant experience in the out of doors," explained a 1955 camp brochure. Armstrong, along with mentor and friend Edmund R. Tomb, Area Executive Secretary, could see the writing on the wall for Wawayanda, so when the opportunity arose to sell the storied camp to neighboring landowner Frederick Hussey III for $500,000, the deal was done in 1954.

Once again, Wawayanda was on the move. As volunteers from the Westfield N.J. YMCA Men's Club dismantled Andover cabins and

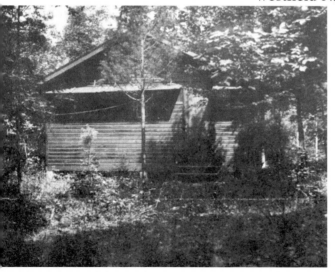

reassembled them at Camp Speers, the CAAC solidified the three-year lease of a small camp owned by Stevens Institute of Technology near Johnsonburg, in adjoining Warren County, New Jersey. The property, 12 miles from Wawayanda, had been developed in the 1930s to provide field training for Stevens' engineering and surveying students. "We rented it for eight weeks each summer with the agreement that we would keep our staff on for two more weeks in September to feed their students," Armstrong explained.

Johnsonburg had a lake, cabins twice the size of Wawayanda's, a dining hall and two rec halls. There were archery and crafts, songs and campfires. The "Trail Blazer" program that provided Adirondack hiking, deep sea fishing, and other more rigorous adventures for older boys had been started in 1954 and was continued at the new camp, where tamer pursuits included chess, nature study and whittling. But former Andover campers who summered there in 1955, '56 and '57 just couldn't summon up much affection for the place. Their memories of the old camp, and their anxiety about the future, colored the Johnsonburg experience, and their memories of it. "We all had strong attachments to Andover, and when it was sold it was kind of unsettling," said Christopher Jones, a Wawayanda camper in the 1940s and a counselor and staff member during the 1950s. Johnsonburg, he recalled, "was a place we landed for a few years, and we tried to maintain some sense of continuity, to carry over what we

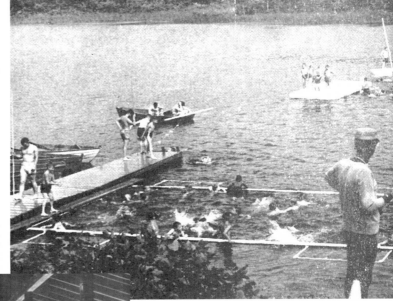

Swimming "Crib" at Johnsonburg

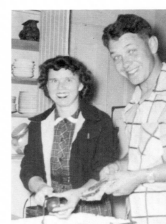

Directors Earl & Bea Armstrong

Dining Hall at Steven's Institue Camp

could from the old camp."

That included the names of the villages (though the Johnsonburg cabins were not arranged in clusters but were instead scattered through the woods); the "W" and Wings awards; and, of course, "Wawayanda Grace." A large drafting room that had been used by Stevens students became the chapel the first summer at Johnsonburg until an outdoor worship site was prepared. Morning worship and evening vespers remained an important part of the daily agenda as Wawayanda emphasized its objective of "developing Christian personality and building a Christian society." During Sunday services, campers and staff contributed to the YMCA's World Service Program, which funded youth development activities in other countries. In 1955, 100 camper hymnals were shown at the top of a list of new equipment, which included four rifles, softball gear, ten backpacks for the Trail Blazers, and a 25-foot "war canoe."

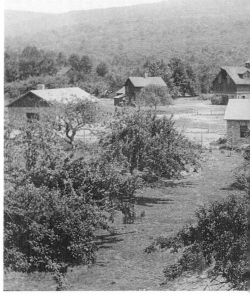

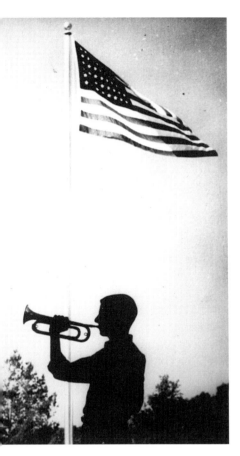

While some things stayed the same (like Campers Day, when campers were elected to act as counselors, camp director and other posts for a day), others were disturbingly different. Jones, who had been camp bugler at Andover, still shudders at the remembered sound of recorded bugle calls broadcast over the Johnsonburg loudspeaker.

Al Chrone, former Andover camper who by the 1950s was on the staff at the Westfield Y, remembers that Johnsonburg's lake had no shallow end, and a special wooden "crib" had to be constructed for swimming, making it undesirable for the Westfield family campers he was trying to recruit. Instead of Johnsonburg, Westfield families went to Delaware for their annual getaway.

But many people did come to Johnsonburg. A Labor Day Family Camping Weekend drew 15 families in 1956, the year 1,745 people attended college, business and church conferences at the site during the off-season. More than 520 boys attended summer camp that year.

But "It just wasn't Camp Wawayanda," said Bud Cox, who was in the Andover dining hall the day Charles R. Scott was stricken in 1954, and went on to spend the next three summers at Johnsonburg. As if to demonstrate that the interim facility didn't quite ring true, the old iron bell that had called thousands of campers to meals at Andover had been transported to Johnsonburg, where it was incorrectly hung and so did not resonate well. To summon campers, the camp cook took to banging on it with a big metal spoon, Chris Jones remembers, and one day it cracked, never to ring again.

Meanwhile, YMCA officials were desperately searching for a permanent home for Wawayanda. In 1956, the stars aligned as two active Y supporters got together to negotiate the purchase of what would become the camp's new base in the Catskill Mountains of New York State.

That's where wool baron Julius Forstmann had established a luxurious summer retreat in the valley of the West Branch of the Neversink River at Branch, N.Y. In 1904 Forstmann had come to America from Germany, where his ancestors had operated a lucrative and well-respected wool manufacturing business. The young immigrant used what he'd learned in the Old Country to set up a mill in Passaic, N.J., and the Forstmann Woolen Company quickly built a reputation for high quality dresswear in the U.S. The company also provided uniforms and combat clothing for American servicemen during both World Wars.

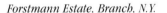

Forstmann Estate, Branch, N.Y.

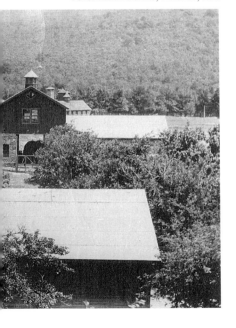

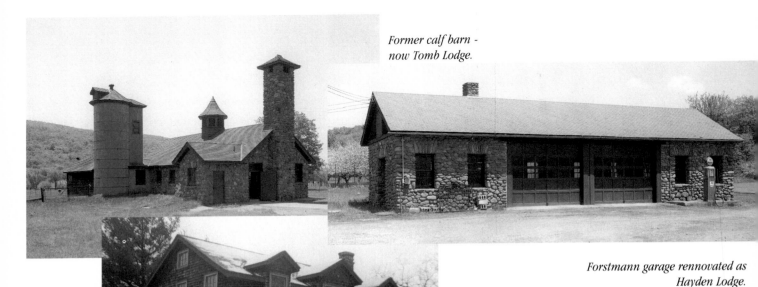

Former calf barn - now Tomb Lodge.

The Carriage House became Biscuit Lodge.

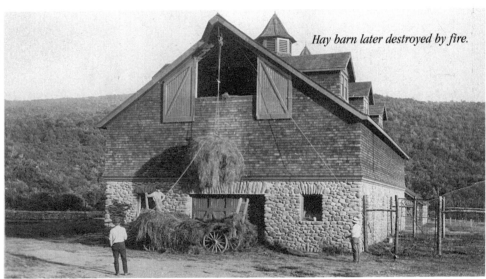

Forstmann garage rennovated as Hayden Lodge.

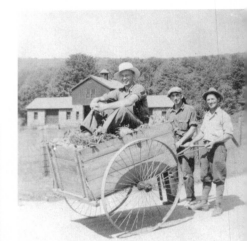

Hay barn later destroyed by fire.

Following a 1914 fishing trip to the Catskills, Julius Forstmann decided to invest some of his wealth in 2,200 acres of exquisite farm and forest land in the Neversink Valley. The scenic vistas and natural resources of this wild land at the intersection of Sullivan and Ulster Counties had long been a magnet for public and private interests. Early settlers had eked a living from rocky, hillside farms. Entrepreneurs had harvested timber, quarried bluestone, stripped hemlock bark for use in tanning leather, and harnessed streams for mills of every description. New York State had acquired thousands of acres of undeveloped land and in 1888 designated them part of the new "forever wild" Catskill Forest Preserve; four years later the first foot trail was blazed to 4,200-foot-tall Slide Mountain, the highest in the Catskills.

Biscuit Brook

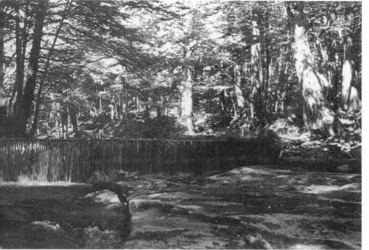

The crystalline water springing from these mountains had long been storied for its purity. Tourists, artists, anglers and writers like naturalist John Burroughs savored the special qualities of the Catskills. The Neversink, wrote Burroughs, "was one of the finest trout streams I had ever fished. . . . It had a new look as though it had just come from the hands of its Creator."

Biscuit Brook, a tributary of the West Branch of the Neversink, meandered through the farm acquired by Julius Forstmann, who spared no effort or expense at building a summer showplace. The estate featured a 23-room, three-story stone and shingle residence, a well-tended dairy farm and beautifully manicured lawns and gardens. Julius and his wife Adolphine brought their five children – Reinhold, Carl, Curt, Julius and Louise – for long, lazy summers spent fishing, riding, and hunting in their 800-acre fenced deer preserve stocked with whitetails from Michigan and the Adirondacks. The family also had homes in Passaic and in New York City, and enjoyed sailing the waters of the world aboard the Orion, their 330-foot-long yacht, the largest in the world, capable of accommodating 232 passengers.

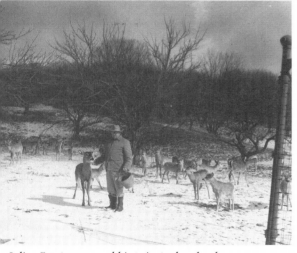

Julius Forstmann and his private deer herd.

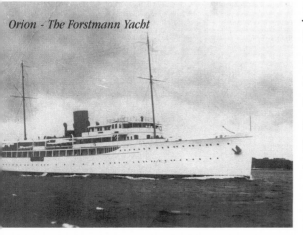

Orion - The Forstmann Yacht

The family's fortunes were not always so rosy, however. Son Carl Forstmann was killed in an auto accident in 1922. Both Julius, the patriarch of the family, and eldest son Reinhold, died in 1939. Son Curt then managed the company and the Catskills estate until he died at age 43 in 1950. Remaining son Julius finally sold the Forstmann Woolen Company to J. P. Stevens and Company in 1957. In 1956, he had let it be known that the family's magnificent Catskill Mountain estate was on the market. The worlds of the Forstmanns and the New Jersey YMCA were about to intersect.

Enter Bernie Forster of Ridgewood, who had been a generous contributor to the Ridgewood Y and a founder of its Camp Bernie. Forster was said to have been a fishing guest of the Forstmanns, and to have contacted another fishing companion, Henry Hird, when he discovered the Forstmann estate was for sale.

Hird was also from Ridgewood, past president and director of the Y there, chairman of the New Jersey State YMCA and of its camping committee. He was the son of Samuel Hird memorialized in the swimming dock at Wawayanda in Andover. Like Julius Forstmann, Samuel Hird had started a woolen manufactory, Samuel Hird and Sons. "I was always told by my father that the senior Julius had given Samuel much advice to help Samuel get started," related Henry's son, H. Edward Hird. "Respect between the next generation of Hirds and Forstmanns continued over the years."

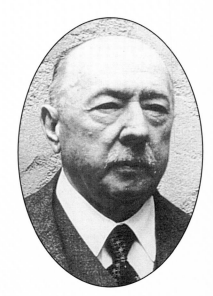

Julius Forstmann

Serving as counsel for the Forstmann business was attorney Walter Margetts, former New Jersey State Treasurer, trustee for the Morristown YMCA, and founder and president of New Jersey Camp for the Blind. The Margetts and Forstmann families were not only business associates but friends; their children played together, and Julius Forstmann the younger was godfather to Margetts' son, Tom.

"We got a call from Henry Hird, chairman of the Wawayanda Camping Committee, saying that the (Forstmann) property was for sale," remembered Earl Armstrong, camping consultant for the CAAC. "Ed Tomb (Area Executive Secretary) and I looked at it, walked over a lot of it, saw the buildings, came back and said 'Let's buy it. We can't afford not to.'"

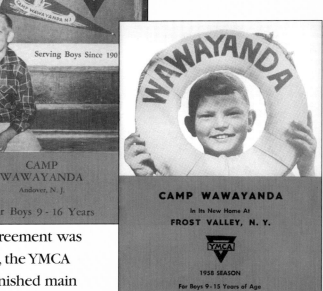

Walter Margetts and Henry Hird were called upon to negotiate the deal with Julius Forstmann, and an agreement was reached Christmas Eve, 1956. At the closing on April 1, 1957, the YMCA paid $130,000 for the 2,200-acre property, including the furnished main house, 12 fully-equipped farm buildings, and a registered herd of 22 Holsteins, 14 heifers and a bull. Some people called it a steal, others a gift that would yield lasting benefits to generations unborn. The Forstmann estate would be preserved, Camp Wawayanda had a new home (albeit in a different state), and the future was rife with possibilities.

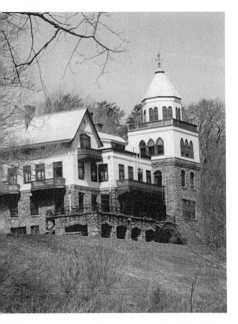

But before transformation of a summer estate to a boys' camp could commence, a new organizational structure had to be effected. The CAAC, wishing to divest itself of camp administration duties, approved the formation of the Frost Valley Association, which would manage and fund operations of Camp Wawayanda and of the envisioned Forstmann Conference and Vacation Center. A board of directors was appointed by the CAAC, and included representatives of the New Jersey YMCAs which would make use of Frost Valley: Bergen County, Eastern Union County, Madison, Montclair, Perth Amboy, Plainfield, Ridgewood, Summit and Westfield. The CAAC also named an executive director of the new enterprise, Ray Grant, who divided his time between CAAC offices in Newark and Frost Valley. Grant had left the executive director's chair at the Westfield Y to take the Frost Valley post. He was succeeded at Westfield by Ed Ewen, former

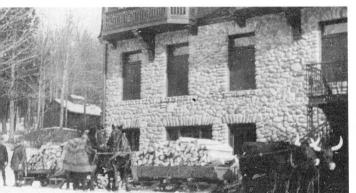

Wawayanda camper and staffer who later joined the Frost Valley board representing one of the key Ys to use the new facility.

Earl Armstrong remained as camp director, and, while camp continued for a third and final year at Johnsonburg, work began at the Frost Valley site. First, with an eye toward producing some income, visiting groups and guests were welcomed at the main house, which came to be known as "The Castle." It provided elegant quarters, with cherry,

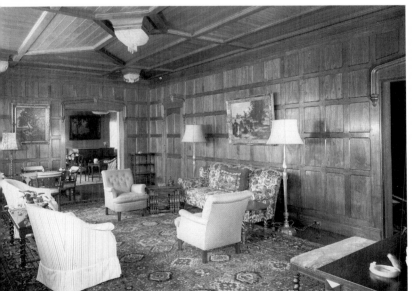

butternut and maple woodwork, teak and oak parquet flooring, seven fireplaces and six baths. Mounted game trophies and handsome antiques decorated the building, including an 18th-century grandfather clock and a Steinway piano on which Adolphine Forstmann reputedly learned to play. A 15x36-foot game room was situated on the third floor, beneath a stone observation tower, where Forstmann children, and later grandchildren, were tutored during the summer months, and where the bravest of them watched lightning flash around them during booming thunder storms.

"Castle Girls" served as hostesses. They prepared food, made beds, polished the brass fixtures and, on slow days, occasionally amused themselves riding up and down on the dumb waiter.

The first Frost Valley campers – 569 of them – arrived in the summer of 1958. A lake was bulldozed from the Castle field. The lake, stagnant and filled with frogs, made for poor swimming that first year.

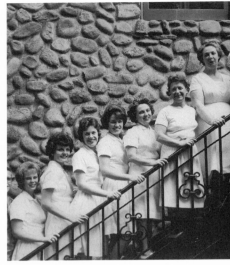

The "Castle Girls"

Earl Armstrong and Henry Hird staked out the cabin sites, and Armstrong designed the cabins. They were hammered together in one of the barns by Harry Cole, who had been the Forstmanns' caretaker and stayed on for several years after the estate's sale to serve as buildings and grounds superintendent at Frost Valley. As soon as the frost left the ground in the spring of 1958, the 25 cabins were raised, but it was up to incoming counselors and staff to apply finishing touches (like roofs and floors) during training week just before camp started that summer.

That first summer, campers and staff ate in the renovated main dairy barn. "It still had the cow stanchions," recalled John Ketcham, a 1958 camper. "Each cabin had its own table in a stanchion."

Camp Director Armstrong recruited the counselors. "We were looking for Number 1, character, and Number 2, experience – people who could carry out the Christian purpose of the YMCA," he explained. Counselors came from all over the country, many from the south. One of them was Dave King, who was hired as Lenape Village Chief while a junior at Towson State Teachers College in Maryland. He was paid $600 for

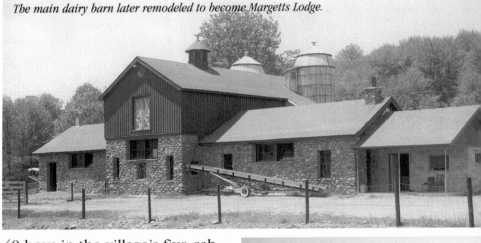

The main dairy barn later remodeled to become Margetts Lodge.

the eight-week season, in charge of 40 boys in the village's five cabins. Other Village Chiefs were King's college-mate Mike DeVita (Forest Village), Merrill Oleson (Totem), Conrad Hawkins (Outpost) and Harry Owen (Hemlock). Some staff members from the Andover years came north to work at Frost Valley. They included waterfront director Hal Ressmyer and riflery instructor Bill McNally. To many young campers, certain staff members were a powerful influence.

Of towering Dave King, John Ketcham recalled, "He was larger than life in many ways. He was exceptional at campfires, and would scare the living daylights out of us with the stories he told. I adored him. But if you crossed him, he'd give you a look that would make

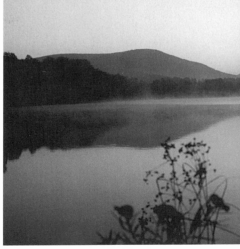

you feel two inches tall." Ketcham would later be a Village Chief himself, under Camp Director Dave King.

Despite the inconveniences, the opening 1958 season was a "great time," according to Earl Armstrong.

The following spring, the 1959 camp booklet, urging families to sign their boys up for two weeks ($85), one month ($170) or a full season ($340), promised that "A 22-acre lake for swimming and boating will be finished before camp opens."

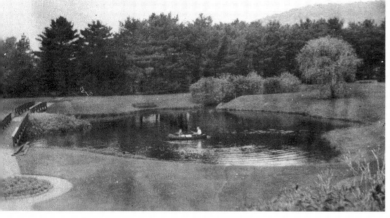

Indeed it was, thanks to the ingenuity of Harry Cole. He built a dam across a swampy area fed by two streams and the West Branch of the Neversink River to create the lake, which was later named for him. He also constructed a new dining hall, later named Thomas Lodge, which had been delivered in prefabricated sections aboard flatbed trucks – without plans or blueprints. "If something didn't work, Harry looked at it meanly and made it work," said Dave King of the versatile and talented Mr. Cole. Again, volunteers, many of them from the Westfield Y, pitched in to help complete the project. The hall, with its large central fireplace, quickly became the principal and much beloved camp gathering place.

Other highlights from the 1959 season were the replacement of the 48-star American flag with a 49-star flag at the Independence Day celebration and the annual Olympics in which campers learned about Brazil, Ethiopia, Ireland, Israel and Korea as well as "host" Italy while participating in a pageant and athletic competitions. Four boys and leader Dick Haines climbed nearby Slide Mountain in 50 minutes, 24 seconds without stopping. And 15 Trail Blazers in five canoes paddled 120 miles down the Hudson River, from Fort Edwards to Poughkeepsie, in a six-day adventure with leader Ian Bastelier.

Finally, when the noise and flurry of the camping season had died away, and the Catskill forest had turned shades of crimson and amber, YMCA leaders, supporters and staff members paused on October 10 to dedicate the completed Camp Wawayanda and Forstmann Conference and Vacation Center.

A new decade, with undreamed-of challenges, and even greater potential, was just around the corner.

It still had the cow stanchions, recalled John Ketcham of the barn turned dining hall. Each cabin had its own table in a stanchion.

Lake Cole

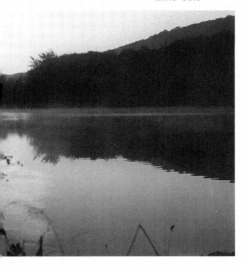

Walter Margetts and Henry Hird

Camp Wawayanda's move from New Jersey to the Catskills could not have happened without Walter T. Margetts, Jr. and Henry E. Hird. On Christmas Eve, 1956, the pair negotiated the transfer of Julius Forstmann's magnificent mountain estate to the Central Atlantic Area Council of the YMCA. Guided by the vision of CAAC Executive Director Edmund R. Tomb, the YMCA paid $130,000 for the 2,200-acre property, including the furnished main house, 12 fully-equipped farm buildings and a herd of Holstein cattle. Pristine trout streams, thick forests and open valley land made the property ideal for what would become Frost Valley. The quiet but determined efforts of Walter Margetts and Henry Hird produced a holiday gift that would yield lasting benefits to generations yet unborn.

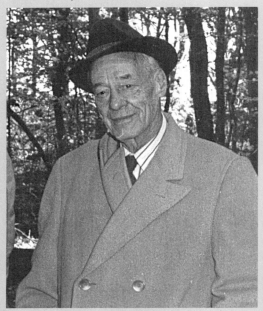

Walter T. Margetts

Attorney Walter T. Margetts (1905-1983), a native of Passaic, was well known and respected as an influential government, business and civic leader in New Jersey. Named to the National War Labor Board in 1942 by President Franklin D. Roosevelt, he served as New Jersey State Treasurer from 1949 to 1954. He was board chairman and trustee of several companies, and president of the Hudson & Manhattan Railroad. But while he had a head for commerce, Walter Margetts had a heart for children, so when the mother of a blind child suggested establishing a summer camp for the visually impaired, he helped found the New Jersey Camp for the Blind in Morris County, serving as its president for 34 years. He was chairman of the Frost Valley Association, too, and in 1976, a newly renovated, multi-purpose building at the center of camp was named Margetts Lodge in his honor.

Henry Edward Hird's life (1884-1983) was marked by devotion to young people. He served as president of the Passaic Boy's Club, chairman of the Ridgewood YMCA, chairman of the New Jersey State YMCA, and a member of the YMCA's International Committee. While heading up the State Y, he pledged to visit every YMCA in New Jersey and was true to his word, speaking at 40 Ys within a three-month period. Mr. Hird's intellect was broad, his enthusiasm for "Boys Work" infectious, his dedication to the YMCA unbounded. The cabins and lodges constructed above Lake Cole during the 1960s for female campers were named Camp Hird in recognition of Henry and wife Rose's lifelong commitment to youth.

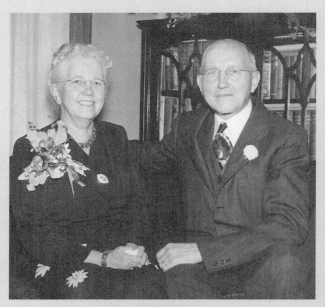

Rose and Henry Hird

Returning to that list of priorities established back in 1961, Brown chose to expand offerings for teenagers. In the summer of 1966, Village Chief Bud Cox had taken a patrol of eight or nine 12- and 13-year-olds on a three-day trek to try to find the wreckage of a small plane that was believed to have crashed on Doubletop Mountain. The Civil Air Patrol hadn't found it, and Bud's campers decided to try. "We bushwhacked through nettles and underbrush from Pigeon Brook," recalled Cox. "Three days in the pouring rain. We never found the plane. I found it fascinating that the kids liked it so much, and it was so miserable."

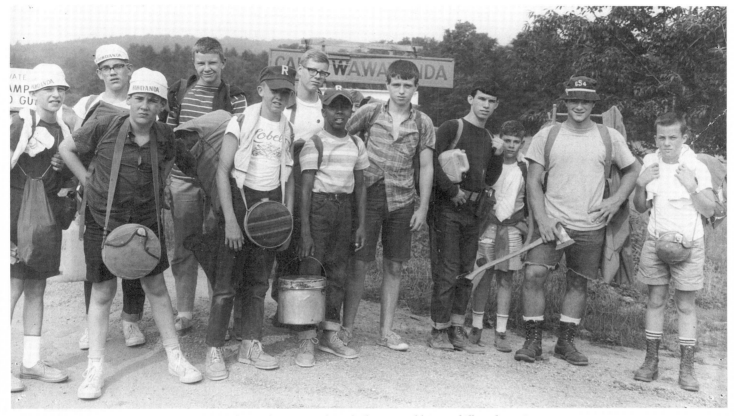

"Bud Cox, (center, rear) with glasses, and his Catskill Explorers"

That was the beginning of Catskill Explorers, a regional backpacking program and the start for many of a lifetime love of the outdoors. Barry Glickman, who later went on to get a degree in outdoor science, work for the US Forest Service and climb mountains, raft rivers, and ski mountain ridges across America, says it all began with Bud Cox. "When I did Slide Mountain all those years ago, it got me hooked on the outdoors," Glickman relates. "With everything that I have done, nothing affects me the way Wawayanda and the Catskills do. Slide means more to me than any other mountain I have ever climbed."

Beyond the Catskills, the Trail Blazers program continued to offer canoe and camping trips to the Adirondacks and Canada. Soon, bike trips throughout the Northeast, Western hiking and canoeing excursions, and other off-campus outings were added to attract adventure-seeking campers. At first, the trips were "boys only" affairs. In 1969, the first co-ed group toured the western states, from Denver to San Francisco.

Frost Valley's building and stretching in the late 1960s came during a period of unrest around the nation. The Vietnam War was raging, the civil rights struggle had led to urban rioting, women were demanding equal treatment at home and in the workplace, and the assassinations of public figures like the Kennedy brothers and Martin Luther King, Jr. had created a backwash of disillusionment in politics and institutions. Where there was not anger, there was apathy.

While some counselors had been "radicalized" on their college campuses and brought these new sensibilities to camp, the broader social turmoil was barely felt at Frost Valley. "I can honestly say I don't remember any discussion of Vietnam at all," conceded Roy Scutro, who came to work as a Wawayanda counselor in 1967. "Frost Valley was not totally isolated, but nobody read the daily newspaper, and TV wasn't available to campers."

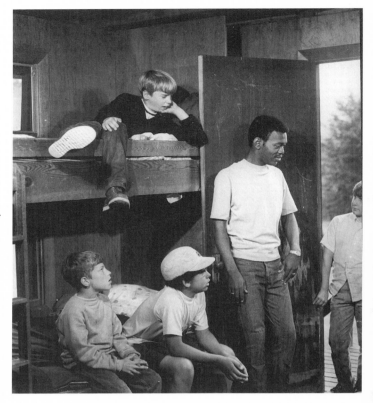

The real world, however, did intrude in a direct and very frightening way, in 1968, when the Newark riots set that city ablaze. As many as 50 campers from Newark were kept at Frost Valley an extra two weeks because it wasn't safe to send them home. Most of them were minority youngsters who'd been sent to camp under a federally-funded program coordinated by the Newark Board of Education. The program later evolved into a cooperative effort among several non-profit service organizations, funded by Victoria Foundation and the Turrell Fund. For 30 years, the Newark Partnership has provided camperships for as many as 140 Newark-area boys and girls each year, allowing city kids to escape the streets and swim in a lake, walk in the woods and lie in a grassy field. The program has sometimes opened the eyes and minds of fellow campers as well.

"The thing he had learned during his two weeks at Frost Valley was that the color of a person's skin does not make a person good or bad."

"I'll never forget the night in Lenape Cabin #20 when a 12-year-old white boy from Ridgewood told his cabinmates and me that he had learned that his father and mother were 'wrong'," recalled former counselor Jim Ewen. "The thing he had learned during his two weeks at Frost Valley was that 'the color of a person's skin does not make a person good or bad.' There were three African-American campers from Newark in his cabin that session."

1968 is also remembered as the year the Frost Valley Association, the interim governing organization of Ys using Frost Valley, was dissolved and Frost

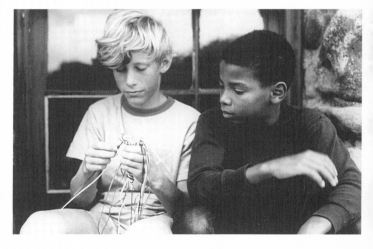

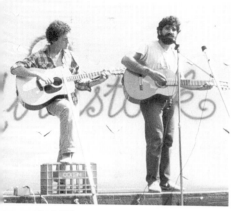

Valley was incorporated as an independent YMCA. "We were standing on our own two feet now. It gave us more flexibility to reach out and serve wider areas, work with additional Ys and other groups," explained Halbe Brown. That year, 763 boys and 560 girls attended Camps Wawayanda and Hird. The numbers were up to 856 boys and 615 girls in 1969.

The 1969 camping season stands out in the memories of the hundreds who lived it. First, there was The Flood. A hurricane that had blown up from the south inundated the Catskills with heavy rains that engorged Biscuit and Pigeon Brooks, changing them from placid creeks to raging torrents. "Biscuit Brook was a brown freight train. It was roaring, a low rumbling roar like no other I have heard before or since," recalled Randy Reed, who was Village Chief of Lenape that year. The water covered the bridge linking the main campus with the Castle and conference facilities, tossed television-sized boulders down the hillsides, and forced all campers and staff into Thomas Lodge. "It rained and rained and rained. Thank God everyone made it to safety," Reed said. "It was a miracle." The experience was a frightening one, but, as with floods before and since, the damage to athletic fields, the waterfront and roadways was repaired and camp continued for the season.

The first manned moon landing transfixed America in July of 1969. Campers assembled outside the Castle to view a small television placed in one of the windows, applauding the successful lunar landing. Later, they staged a capsule re-entry "re-enactment," firing a flaming arrow into the lake, where divers escorted a canoe carrying three counselors in jumpsuits to shore and a waiting "NASA" van.

And then there was the Woodstock Music and Art Fair on Max Yasgur's farm in Bethel, Sullivan County, just 20 miles, as the crow flies, from Frost Valley. To feel a part of "three days of peace and music," Frost Valley campers and counselors staged "Hirdstock," a festival of home-grown talent that became an annual event.

This was a time when Ys everywhere were re-examining their programs in an effort to remain relevant and engaged. As the decade rolled to a close in 1969, Frost Valley launched a new initiative that would prove to be both. An Environmental Education Center had not been envisioned in the "Grand Design" of 1961, but its mission was

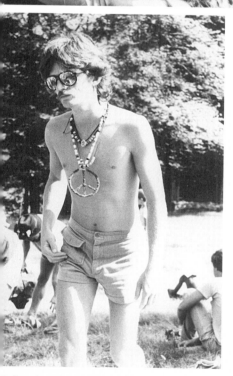

irdstock - Frost Valley's answer to Woodstock

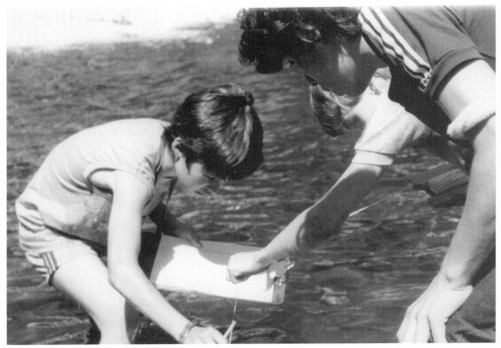

The stream becomes the classroom.

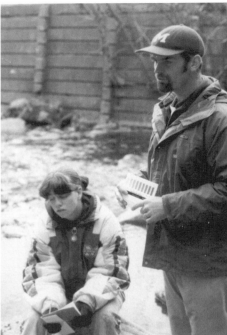

David Scherf, right, teaches water ecology.

one that resonated with teachers, students and individuals concerned about the health of the planet. One year before the first annual Earth Day raised global consciousness about the effects of pollution on air, land and water, Frost Valley established a year-round center to introduce young people to the natural world and show them how to protect it.

The center was directed by Bill Devlin. The former property manager for the Philadelphia Girl Scouts, Devlin held a similar position at Frost Valley. Resident Director when Halbe Brown was in New Jersey during the off-season, Devlin managed the office, repaired frozen water lines, and even drove to Kingston every Thursday to buy food for weekend guests and groups. Always searching for a way to keep the budget balanced, Brown and Devlin decided to look into the relatively new field of outdoor, or environmental education. With assistance from Nassau County BOCES on Long Island, which provided advice, funding and interested schools, Frost Valley launched the program that would make further use of the facility.

Near at hand were all the resources for programs on ferns and fungi, geology, pond and stream life, astronomy and more. Sixteen schools brought groups to the valley during the center's first year. Students and teachers stayed in winterized buildings during fall, winter and spring visits, studying native plants, following wildlife tracks and observing seasonal changes to mountain habitats. Teachers ran their own programs with guidance from a manual Devlin developed, and from college interns who worked at Frost Valley in exchange for course credit, field work opportunities and room and board.

One college assistant described Devlin as "a radical ethical model – if you did anything wrong, he would just look at you and you confessed immediately. He had a personal relationship with every teacher, and, more than teaching kids about nature, he wanted them to use the opportunity to really get to know their teacher and each other."

Within a few years, as many as 3,000 students were attending the program annually. Environmental Education and Frost Valley were becoming synonymous. During the 1970s, the program would prove itself a crucial part of the expanding Frost Valley universe.

Chapter 6

The '70s – Expanding Possibilities

If the previous decade had begun with Frost Valley searching for direction, the 1970s got underway with its people and programs headed down many exciting paths.

In 1970, Frost Valley was coordinating the International Camper Exchange for the Mid-Atlantic YMCAs, sending boys and girls to Denmark, Germany, Sweden and the Netherlands. Counselors from abroad were also adding to the cultural mix at Frost Valley. By the end of the decade, those programs, and a firm collaboration with the Tokyo YMCA, helped designate Frost Valley as an International YMCA, a leader in cross-cultural initiatives.

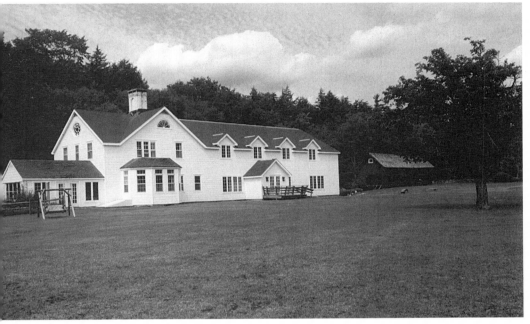

Straus Center

In 1970, the environmental education program was still in its infancy. By 1978, it was offering schools a choice of some 25 programs and had begun to merge some of its lessons with new forest management efforts.

Developing hand-in-hand with the environmental program was Frost Valley's wellness initiative, which proved that good health is a product of informed choices, and that summer camp is a great place to start making them.

In 1970, Frost Valley was reaching out to new audiences to fill the Forstmann Conference Center, and was encouraging the off-season use of its vast acreage by hunters, fishermen and snowmobilers. By the end of the decade, it had added a new conference center, attracted hordes of cross-country skiers and had doubled its land holdings with the acquisition of the Straus and Tison estates.

And in a decade marked by extraordinary developments, among the most notable was the launch, in 1975, of the Ruth Carole Gottscho Dialysis Center, the first of its kind anywhere in the world, offering state-of-the-art medical care for children whose kidney disease had heretofore kept them tethered to clinics and hospitals and apart from the beauty, friends and fun that other kids found at summer camp.

"Our hearts were talking to each other."

The establishment of the Ruth Carole Gottscho Dialysis Center at Frost Valley was a huge and risky undertaking. Nowhere else had a sophisticated medical center, with complex equipment and highly trained doctors and nurses, been established in a remote site like Frost Valley, where storms resulted in periodic power outages, the nearest hospital is 25 miles away, and the closest hospital with pediatric dialysis facilities is 130 miles distant. While camps had been created exclusively for children with chronic conditions like asthma, hemophilia and diabetes mellitus, few offered the opportunity for children with special needs to live and play with healthy peers.

That's what Eva Gottscho had hoped for her daughter. Born with malformed kidneys in 1945, at a time when kidney failure was untreatable, Ruth Carole Gottscho spent much of her life in pain and disappointment. "I remember her girl friends would come by the house once school got out and say, 'We're off to summer camp, we'll send you a postcard.' And Ruth would go upstairs and close the door to her room. It was a very sad time in my life and hers," recalled her mother. It was while attempting some therapeutic horseback riding in 1960 that Ruth was thrown from her mount. She went into shock from which she never recovered and died at the age of 15.

It was only after Ruth's death that Eva and her husband Ira

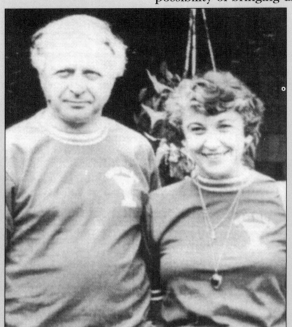
Dr. Ira Greifer and Eva Gottscho

Gottscho heard about long-term dialysis as a means of saving patients awaiting kidney transplantation. The Gottschos, along with a few dedicated friends, established the foundation bearing their daughter's name to raise funds to promote the development of the new technology and make it available to as many patients as possible. Ira Gottscho died in 1971, but Eva and the Foundation carried on, and soon began exploring the possibility of bringing dialysis to a summer camp.

"Nobody wanted us," Eva Gottscho related. "They didn't want to change the food, they didn't want sick kids, they were afraid it would upset the camp. We finally found Frost Valley. We met a few times to talk about it, and at the third meeting, someone from Frost Valley said, 'We're in the business of helping kids. So if you're willing to work with us, we'll work with you.' I don't think we ever had anything in writing. Our hearts were talking to each other. If we'd scoured the world, I don't think we'd have found a better marriage."

Working with the Pediatric Nephrology Unit of the Albert Einstein College of Medicine and the National Association of Patients on Hemodialysis and Transplants, the Gottscho Foundation funded the construction of a $30,000 addition to Smith Lodge, Frost Valley's Health Center. The center featured five hemodialysis machines, a crash cart with resuscitation equipment and medication, an ECG machine and a cardiac monitor-defibrillator. An emergency generator was installed, and a laboratory set up. Physicians and nurses from the New

The year after the dialysis center was established, another big project was completed. The former main barn of the Forstmann estate, where the first campers in 1958 had eaten among the cow stanchions, was renovated as the multi-purpose Margetts Lodge. The building was stripped of all but its one-story cobblestone base, and was resurrected to include a recreation room (Turrell Hall), two classroom activity centers, and upstairs sleeping quarters for 16 to 24 people. A library was added later. The lodge, dedicated in July of 1976, was named for Walter T. Margetts, Jr., the former chairman of the YMCA Frost Valley Association who played a pivotal role in the Y's acquisition of the Forstmann property.

Chuck White, director of maintenance and development projects, supervised the Margetts reconstruction. He had signed on with Frost Valley in 1973 searching for a less frenetic lifestyle than the one he and wife Joy and their children had in New Jersey. With 25 years in the electronics industry, and a gift for understanding mechanical systems, Chuck secured his new job when, during the interview, he fixed a pitching machine and rewired a haywagon. Over the next 17 years, he designed, coordinated and/or helped construct Frost Valley's new and improved buildings, including, in the 1970s, the Dialysis

York City, New Jersey and Philadelphia areas served as advisors on the project and worked with the young campers at Frost Valley.

Dr. Ira Greifer, Medical Director of the National Kidney Foundation and Director of Einstein's pediatric nephrology unit, was instrumental in cutting through the red tape in two states to set up the camp center. Dr. William Primack of Einstein, and Sheryl Melber, a Detroit nurse, were the first operating coordinators of the unit. Nurses Michele Palamidy and Stuart Kaufer later had supervisory roles. Dr. Frederick J. Kaskel was one of the first physicians to work at the Gottscho Center. Now the Director of the Division of Pediatric Medicine at the Ira Greifer Children's Kidney Center at Montefiore Hospital, he continues to play a leadership role in the Frost Valley facility.

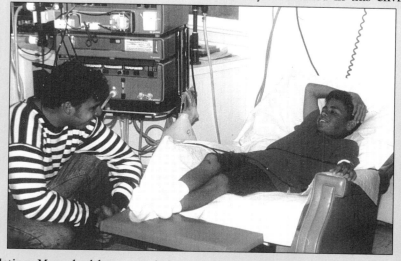

There were 22 children in four camp sessions that first summer, the cost of their camp stay and treatment covered by the Foundation. Many had been on dialysis for 18 months or longer, meaning they had been hooked to a blood-cleansing machine two to three times a week, for four to six hours each time. Twelve of them were unsuccessful transplant patients. All had been stunted and scarred, physically, emotionally and socially.

Frost Valley provided the antidote. The kids had their blood pressure monitored and medications dispensed daily at the center. Dialysis was conducted every other day and was scheduled to allow the children to participate in regular camp activities as much as possible. They enjoyed dinner and nighttime socializing with other cabinmates. The camp menu was modified for dialysis patients when necessary, and counselors were trained in aspects of their condition and treatment. Fellow campers and counselors were encouraged to visit during dialysis, so the center was often a place of songs, crafts, books and games. The rest of the time, dialysis campers swam, rode horses, learned archery and all the rest.

They blossomed in this environment of acceptance and challenge. One fragile-seeming Bronx boy who had come to camp dependent on a walker, refused to take it home with him and left it at Frost Valley, where he had discovered he could navigate without it. "These kids were funny, intuitive, and won everyone over," said Al Filreis, camp program director from 1975 to 1978. "They were stars. I don't think anyone anticipated that aspect of the program. It was really something to see the tears of joy on the faces of parents as they saw their children hugging new friends, and exchanging addresses and phone numbers."

It has worked this way for more than 25 years now. Counselors, too, who are kidney patients have been able to integrate their jobs with treatment. They may not be able to take a vacation from their illness, but for two weeks, kidney patients can participate in the simple joys of summer camp while their families experience a respite from continuous care and worry.

Center; the fire house constructed as a substation of the Claryville Fire Dept.; and renovations to the newly-acquired Straus estate. He also supervised construction of the director's residence, built because increasing year-round programming demanded a full-time, on-site director. "Every day was Saturday – I loved to come to work. There was something new to do and think about every day," recalls White.

Joy White served as camp nurse; the White's children helped their father in the maintenance department; daughter Elizabeth taught wilderness survival and "leave no trace" camping to Frost Valley counselors. The Whites, who helped raise 11 foster children, are remembered for the open door and the ready welcome that was always extended for counselors and other staff.

The new Margetts Lodge became the home of the Environmental Education Program. Its director, James Marion, had succeeded Bill Devlin, who had left to become executive director of YMCA Camp Jewell in Connecticut. Marion, a former 4-H youth agent in Sullivan County, arrived in 1976, when he and five or six staff members offered astronomy, planting for wildlife, study of the Eastern bluebird, and trout ecology classes to school groups. "Sensory Night Hikes" and "Under Your Feet" examinations were conducted on a one-mile nature trail, built by Marion as a memorial to Carl Egner, a close friend of Frost Valley Board President Woody English and a long time supporter of youth programs.

In 1978, Marion developed a manual of study programs, augmented by outdoor education adventures like canoeing and rock climbing. With newly-hired educator and forester Mike Larison, a forest clear-cut demonstration plot was established on Middle Mountain to show students how woodlands regenerate. That was the beginning of Frost Valley's Forest Management Program and of serious scientific examination of its own natural resources. Such research would, in the coming years, be shared with learners of all ages. Environmental education was becoming much more than nature study.

"As the twig is bent so grows the tree" was an adage used to describe the "Personal Improvement Project (PIP)" initiated by Frost Valley Physician Dr. William Hettler in 1976. Health Services Director at the University of Wisconsin, Stevens Point, Dr. Hettler started with the premise that it's easier to develop a healthy lifestyle as a young person, than to change a damaging one as an adult. Eleven- and 12-year-old campers planned and prepared various diets, tested the physical effects of sports and activities, analyzed samples from protected and unprotected waters, and used microscopes to examine dissected sections of animal lungs. Some staff members who were smokers even volunteered as study subjects to determine the effects of their habit.

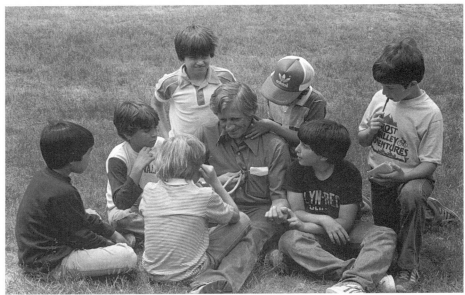

Chuck White gets a checkup from campers in the Wellness Program.

Claudia Swain and camper prepare to embark on The Fitness Trail named for Dr. Jerome Wolff.

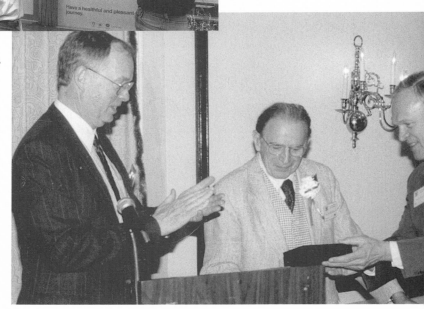

Dr. Jerome Wolff receives the H. R. Quirk Oustanding Volunteer Award from Paul Guenther and Halbe Brown at the 1998 Annual Meeting.

Dr. Hettler's campaign extended to the removal of candy, ice cream and soda from the camp canteen, and to get parents to refrain from stashing sweets in "care" packages from home. Dr. Hettler and Camp Director Mike Ketcham then set out to remove hotdogs, sugary "bug juice," greasy fried rice and other fatty, salty foods from the dining hall menu.

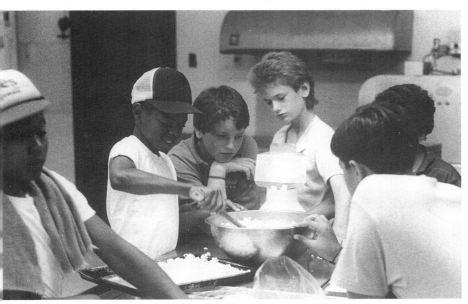

The first salad bar met with puzzled resistance from campers and staff. Counselors took to bringing cupcakes and donuts back from forays to Katz's Bakery in Liberty to give to their campers. A "black market" in candy and soda sprang up. "It was complete chaos for about five years as we adjusted to wellness," quipped Al Filreis, the Program Director for the second half of the decade. "We were a little ahead of the curve, but it was a slow revolution."

Eventually, though, counselors and other staff quit smoking, took up jogging; some even turned to vegetarianism. By 1978 and '79 camp promotional materials described Frost Valley as a place "Where Feeling Good Means Having Fun," a place where prospective campers could "Grow a Lifestyle This Summer." The Camp Log, given to campers to record observations and information about friends and activities, provided space for "Thoughts About Smoking" and "Handling Stress." The Counselors' Manual emphasized ways to introduce the wellness theme within the camp and cabin setting. And the "Incredible Edible" program was set up to allow kids to learn about healthy eating and make treats like banana oatmeal cookies and bran muffins. The low-fat, low sugar philosophy was echoed in the camps' dining halls. In 1980, Mike Ketcham authored and Frost Valley published "Building Wellness Lifestyles" featuring the new wisdom on food, fitness and good health.

The cross country skiing craze burst upon the Frost Valley scene in the mid-1970s, and the camp's rolling valley land, wooded hillsides and streamside corridors proved perfect terrain for ski trails. In 1975, 3,385 conference participants and day visitors were counted as using the trails; by 1978, the number had grown to 10,431.

During spring and fall, fathers and sons came to camp for Y-Indian Guide outings. Begun in 1926 in St. Louis to foster the companionship between fathers and sons, the program's guiding tenets were to "love the sacred circle of my family . . . and to seek and preserve the beauty of the Great Spirit's work in forest, field and stream." In 1971, the Indian Princess program was established for fathers and daughters.

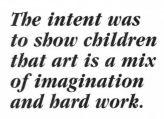

One young Indian Guide, Neil Jordan of Montclair, N.J., became an example to fellow guides and parents as he drank deeply of outdoor fun and comradeship even as he battled leukemia. Neil died in May of 1979, and was memorialized in a totem pole created and carved by Rutgers Art Department Chairman and camp staff member John Giannotti, and erected that summer at the entrance to Frost Valley.

The intent was to show children that art is a mix of imagination and hard work.

The Indian theme reached its zenith in regular camp when Leon VanHeusen, the retired youth and camp director of the Kingston YMCA, brought his fascination and knowledge of Native American cultures to camp. "Van" developed Lacota Indian Village, a replica of a Sioux village where co-ed campers lived in seven 24-foot diameter teepees, met around a council ring, and learned to make totem poles, pack baskets, drums and stone axes. They made moccasins and pipes, maintained a garden, prepared Indian foods, and learned dancing, weather forecasting and language. A camp staff member drove all the way to South Dakota for authentic lodge pole pine logs to build the teepees, and some campers helped strip the bark before the shelters were raised. The village was a busy and popular place for a time, but VanHeusen's sudden death in 1978 took some of the heart out of the project. It carried on for a few years under the able leadership of David Gansler, but was ultimately discontinued.

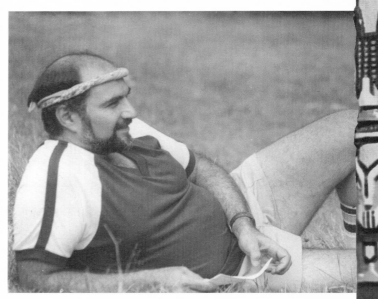

John Giannotti and the totem pole he carved for the entrance to Frost Valley.

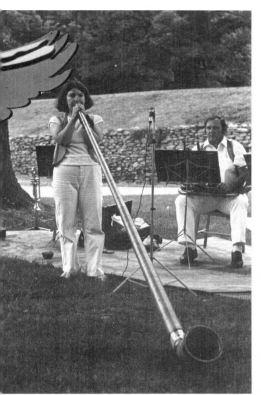

However, 1978 saw the birth of another new summer camp program – Artists-in-Residence. As many as 35 professional sculptors, painters, dancers, singers, musicians, writers and actresses spent three to six days working and living at camp each summer for several years. Poetry and chamber music were thus added to the symphony of camp sounds. John Giannotti said the intent was to show children that art is a mix of imagination and hard work. The special energy and excitement generated by the arts, he said, "help brighten a child's face, and perhaps a child's outlook on life." A special arts village for young people wishing to immerse themselves in creative pursuits was established and named Iscusfa, a Russian word meaning "the arts." A summer Sunday series of concerts and cultural programs was instituted, as was a summer arts week called "Living the Lively Arts," which offered adults the chance to explore photography, traditional music, weaving, drawing, pottery and other artistic pursuits.

Carol Corbin, voice instructor at Rutgers University and Coordinator for the Arts at Frost Valley, was instrumental in implementing these programs. She and architect husband John, also a vocalist, are credited with making the arts an integral facet of Frost Valley life.

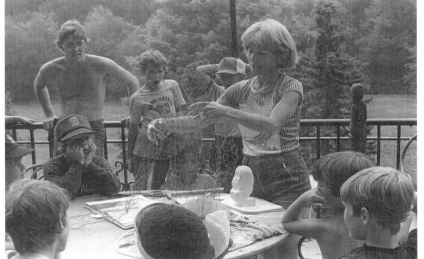

Jody Ketcham begins a wire sculpture; above, Barbara Oldham plays the Alpine horn.

Creativity – and patience and tenacity and empathy – have always been qualities demanded of counselors, particularly those responsible for campers on adventure trips. Jody Davies Ketcham led several such excursions, biking in Maine, rafting in Pennsylvania, glacier climbing in Montana. "Frost Valley gave me the opportunity to be challenged by doing 10,000 things at once," Ketcham said. "We had to be mother, father, craft leader, musician, teacher, psychologist, nurse. All the time, it never stopped."

Capable young staff members were also encouraged to take on responsibility and step into leadership roles. Leslie Black, an avowed "horse nut," remembers that Girls Camp Director Margaret Kremer, forced to fill some unexpected vacancies, elevated her from junior counselor to riding program assistant to riding director in a single summer. "I was 16 years old," Black related. "It was so wonderful, I can't explain. Where else on earth would people believe in you so much?"

Many teens were given the opportunity to explore Europe through the YMCA's International Camper Exchange Program, which began in 1962 when a connection was made between Wawayanda's brother camp Dudley and a Y camp in Germany. Frost Valley became involved in the program in the late 1960s, sending campers abroad and hosting foreign campers. Young people spent a month traveling to selected YMCA host camps in several countries. The International Camp Counselor Program also placed counselors in participating Y camps. College students from the Middle East, Africa, Europe, South America and Asia brought the world to the Neversink Valley. Both programs continue today, spreading global goodwill and understanding through person-to-person contact.

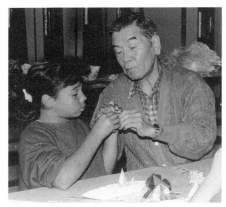

The art of Origami

The Y's international work expanded in 1979 with the signing of the Tokyo-New York YMCA Partnership agreement. Spawned at a "Japan Night" in New York City as the Tokyo YMCA was planning its centennial celebration, the Partnership was intended to help the estimated 50,000 Japanese nationals who were assigned temporarily to jobs at several hundred Japanese corporations in the metropolitan area. "The purpose was to help Japanese youth and family have a meaningful time while they stayed in this country, and to build greater understanding between the two countries," explained Emiko Honma, whose husband Tatsuo Honma was re-assigned from his duties as executive director of the Central Tokyo YMCA to direct the new Partnership program in the U.S.

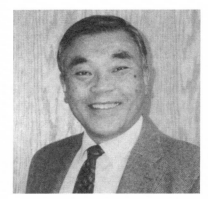

Tatsuo Honma

For the first three years, the program sent Japanese children to summer camp at Holiday Hills, the camp and conference center of the YMCA of Greater New York. But the facilities were quickly outgrown. In 1982, the Partnership found Frost Valley, and split its camp offerings between the two facilities, where Japanese youth played, made friends and studied Japanese culture and language with their peers in the relaxed atmosphere of summer camp. The program grew to include sports camps, twice-yearly ski camps, and by 1991, when the exclusive Frost Valley Partnership was formalized, 1,000 people were participating in summer and winter camp activities. The program offices were located at Frost Valley, and the Partnership employed five year-round and 45 summer staff people. Today, 3,000 people participate in Partnership activities each year, and 400 campers experience Frost Valley through the program.

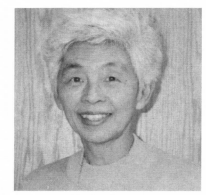

Emiko Honma

"Nobody expected it to grow like this," said Emiko Honma, "but

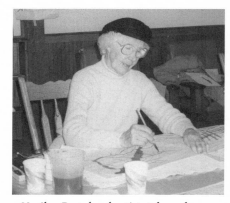

Marilyn Barr, local artist, takes a lesson in Japanese brush work.

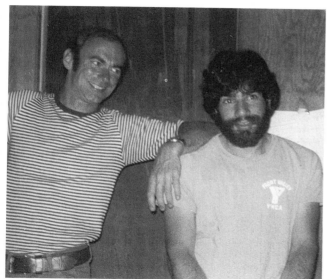

Michael Ketcham and Al Filreis

we were determined, and Frost Valley people were so understanding." The Honmas directed the program for 18 years, and helped develop Friendship House at Frost Valley, a permanent tribute to the Partnership (see Chapter 8).

In 1979, Frost Valley appointed its first full-time, year-round Director of Camping, Michael Davidson Ketcham, who took over the job of coordinating both Camps Wawayanda and Hird, giving Executive Director Halbe Brown more time to devote to the overall operation of Frost Valley. A former camper hailing from a Westfield, N.J. family long active in the YMCA, Ketcham had also been a counselor at Frost Valley, leading several Western Adventure trips. A graduate of the London School of Economics, former Naval officer and high school teacher, he returned to Frost Valley where he found an enthusiastic "sidekick" in Al Filreis, then director of Wawayanda.

The two men made it a practice to walk through each boys' camp village every evening, visiting every cabin. "We used pillow fluffing as an excuse to get near each kid, to wish them goodnight, to hear them talk softly to each other, to make sure they were alright, especially the young ones," said Filreis. "But even the cool 15-year-old boys loved it. They'd compete to see whose pillow would get fluffed first."

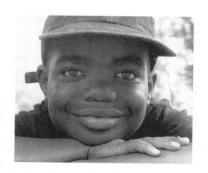

As the decade closed, Frost Valley was like a growing oak with ever-spreading branches, and summer camp was its sturdy trunk. An experiment in centralization that had largely shifted authority for programing and governance from Village Chiefs to the camp directors had been abandoned in 1976. "We'd lost the village control that made camp seem smaller than it was, where the village chief was the 'local governor' of a small cluster of cabins, and where what happened in one village was different than any other, based on the skills, attitudes and personalities of the chiefs and counselors," remembered Al Filreis.

That loss of intimacy and distinctiveness, and the unwieldy nature of the centralized system, prompted Executive Director Halbe Brown to return to the village-based concept that had proved so successful when it was introduced to Wawayanda by director John Ledlie in the 1930s. It gave village chiefs more responsibility, authority and latitude, and restored Ledlie's time-tested legacy.

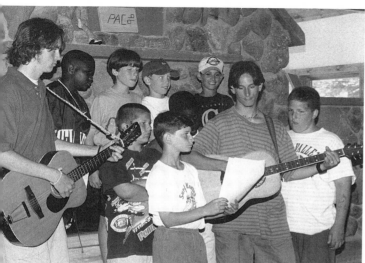

Frost Valley talent show

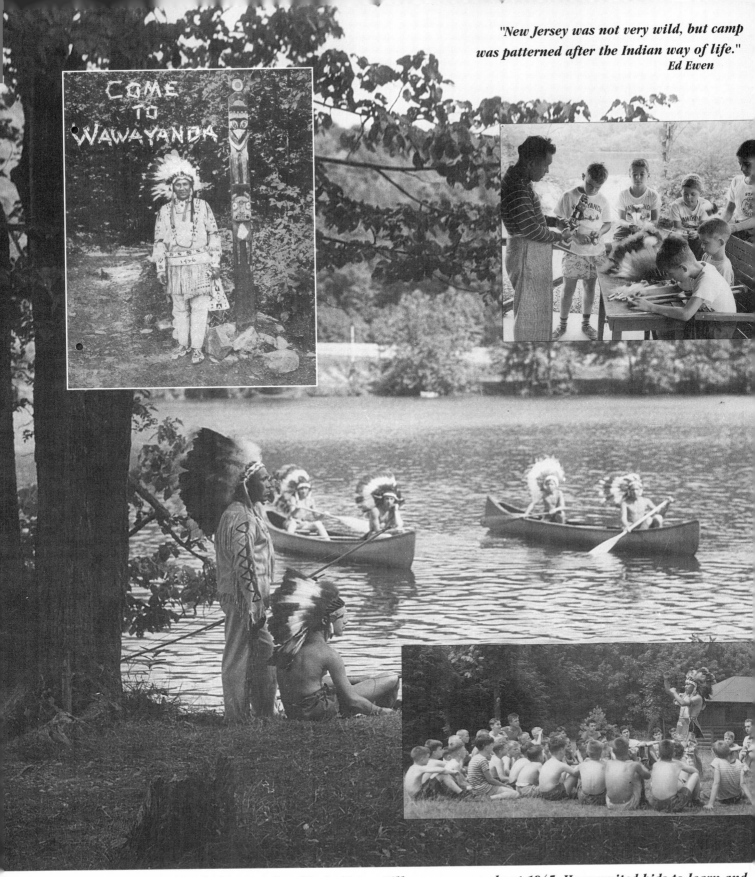

"New Jersey was not very wild, but camp was patterned after the Indian way of life."
Ed Ewen

COME TO WAWAYANDA

"I was a camper in Chief White Bear's cabin in Totem Village one year, about 1945. He recruited kids to learn and participate in an Indian dance, which was the evening program at the main council ring by Indian Rock in the woods. I remember learning the steps and dressing in Indian costume. The dance had something to do with dogs, because we were supposed to bark. Chief White Bear also had a drum with a leather head and Indian designs on it. He offered it up for sale, so I bought it and kept it for years." Chris Jones

INDIAN WAYS

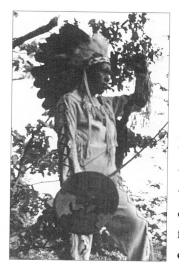

Native American themes – respect for the earth, creation of artful and utilitarian objects from natural resources, and a basic spirituality – were made to order for the camp setting. At Wawayanda in Andover, a totem pole was carved and erected at the entrance to Totem Village; tom toms were made in craft class, "war canoes" were sailed on the lake, and bracelets with Indian heads were created in metal shop. Chief White Bear was a counselor at Wawayanda in Andover. Reputed to be a full-blooded Native American, he taught Indian lore at camp, and at area schools and YMCAs for several years. Many Wawayanda campers, while they cannot recall the Chief's full name or his tribal affiliation, retain vivid memories of White Bear: The Indian symbols he painted on dining hall tables and on the hall's ceilings; the traditional songs and stories he taught them; how he would paint their names in Indian signs on their raincoats. "It was something of a status symbol," Ted Jackson recalled.

Lacota Village resurrected the theme, complete with teepees and craft classes, at Frost Valley in the 1970s.

During spring and fall, fathers and sons came to camp for Y-Indian Guide outings. Begun in 1926 in St. Louis to foster the companionship between fathers and sons, the program's guiding tenets were to "love the sacred circle of my family . . . and to seek and preserve the beauty of the Great Spirit's work in forest, field and stream." In 1971, the Indian Princess program was established for fathers and daughters.

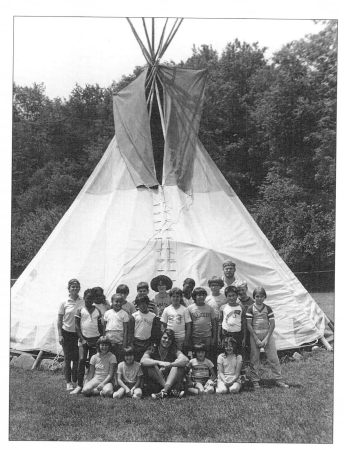

Lacota Village

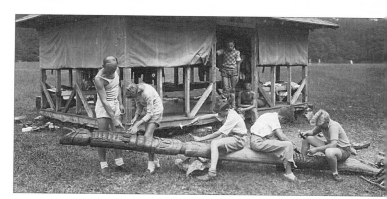

Totem carving

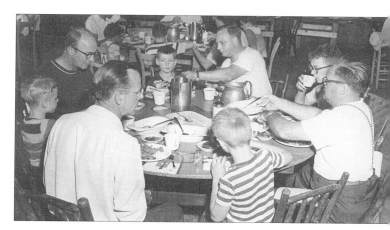

Indian Guides

Music – around a campfire, in the dining hall, at lakeside ceremonies – has always been a signature of summer camp at Wawayanda and Frost Valley. From hymns sung at morning vespers, to "Wawayanda Grace" at meals, to "Taps" intoned by a bugler at dusk, the moments of a camper's day has traditionally been punctuated by song.

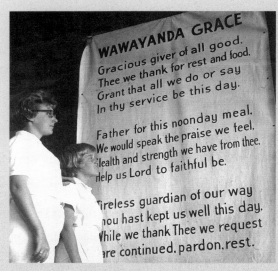

WAWAYANDA GRACE
Gracious giver of all good,
Thee we thank for rest and food,
Grant that all we do or say
In thy service be this day.

Father for this noonday meal,
We would speak the praise we feel,
Health and strength we have from thee,
Help us Lord to faithful be.

Tireless guardian of our way
Thou hast kept us well this day,
While we thank Thee we request
Are continued, pardon, rest.

"Wawayanda was practically founded on music, for, on the first day of the first camping season, 'Uncle Ed' (Edwin) Beach of Orange presented a small folding organ to the camp," wrote Hugh P. Scott in a *Wawayanda Whirlwind* from the 19-teens. "William J. Harris of Verona was our next musical sponsor, his contribution being an old-fashioned square piano. George Hogeman, Joseph N. Brown, Lew F. Cronk, Judson Drayton, Arthur Wilson, Alfred Peil and Randolph Merrill were among early accompanists who presided at the keyboard. . . Gathered round them, campers joined heartily in singing patriotic, college, camp, folk and sacred music which floated across island-dotted waters to echo from fringing forests."

In the age before radio and television, camp music was often far more than the sing-along variety. The

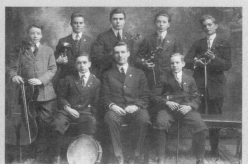

1915 Farewell Dinner at Wawayanda was a formal affair at which the eight-member Wawayanda Orchestra (four violins, a piano, a violincello, a cornet and drums) performed the "Panama Pacific" march and the Overture from "Lucia di Lammermoor." A quartet also entertained, and campers sang "Wawayanda Grace" and "Wawayanda All Along the Line".

Concerts and musical productions have been staged by campers and counselors over the years. At the camp's second home near Andover, N.J., the "Wawayanda Opera House" was the scene of several shows each season. In 1939, the Wawayanda Players staged a radio play, a minstrel show, a stunt night and an ambitious musical, "The Conquistador," about South American liberator Simon Bolivar. "Show Boat" was the big production in 1950. Val Meinzer and Paul "Rugged" Dimitriades produced, directed and acted in the show, which also starred Jack Dell, Jim Waite and Gaylord Ravenal.

"A Singing Camp is a Happy Camp" asserted an article in the camp newsletter in July of 1960, when Mike "Perry" DeVita put out a call for voices for the re-activated Wawayanda Choir.

Whether organized or informal, music made an indelible impression on many campers and counselors. "I remember the singing," recalled Jim Ewen, "the songs during the late '60s and '70s focusing on the need for peace, justice and harmony in our world. It made a huge impact on me, it shaped many of my values and beliefs."

David Sunshine, a camper and staff member in the 1970s and '80s, also cherishes his musical Frost Valley memories. Now a music teacher in Maryland, he has spent recent summers as a Frost Valley artist-in-residence, leading songfests, serenading dialysis campers, performing at special events. As part of his crusade to reinforce and encourage the singing tradition at Frost Valley, Sunshine compiled the lyrics to dozens of traditional and contemporary camp songs. They range from gospel standards like "Do Lord" and "Amazing Grace", to Woody Guthrie's classic "This Land," to anti-war anthems like Bob Dylan's "Blowin' in the Wind." Silly songs, too, make up the camp repertoire, tunes like "Do Your Ears Hang Low," "Dead Skunk," "Prune Song" and the "Announcements Song" ("A terrible death to be talked to death, a terrible death to die. . .").

WAWAYANDA WATERS.

F. F. G.

Frank F. Gray.

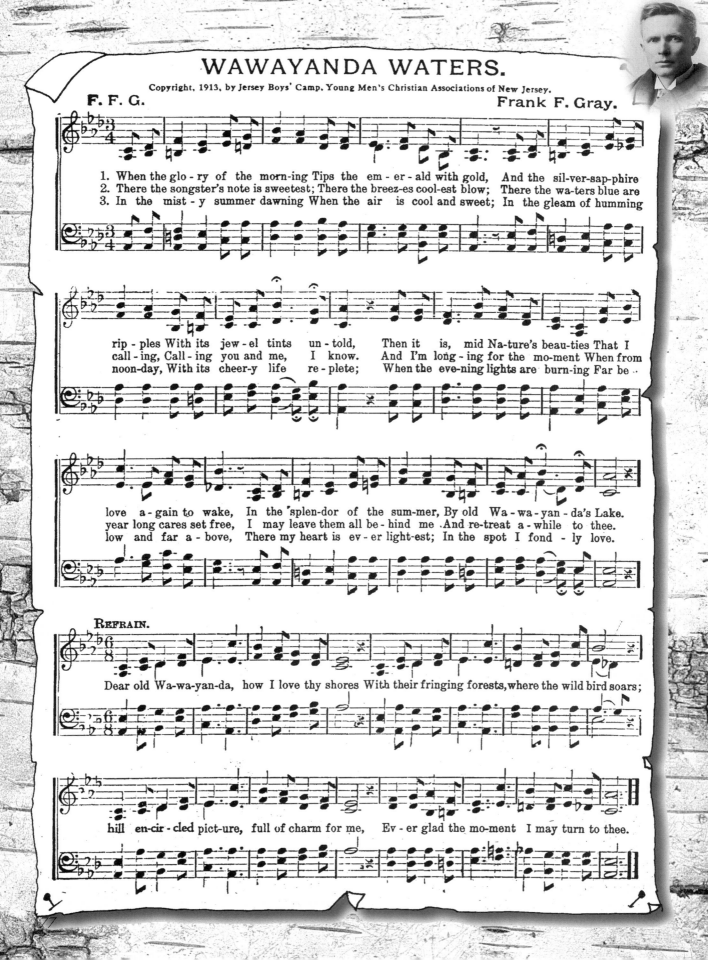

1. When the glo-ry of the morn-ing Tips the em-er-ald with gold, And the sil-ver-sap-phire
2. There the songster's note is sweetest; There the breez-es cool-est blow; There the wa-ters blue are
3. In the mist-y summer dawning When the air is cool and sweet; In the gleam of humming

rip-ples With its jew-el tints un-told, Then it is, mid Na-ture's beau-ties That I
call-ing, Call-ing you and me, I know. And I'm long-ing for the mo-ment When from
noon-day, With its cheer-y life re-plete; When the eve-ning lights are burn-ing Far be-

love a-gain to wake, In the 'splen-dor of the sum-mer, By old Wa-wa-yan-da's Lake.
year long cares set free, I may leave them all be-hind me And re-treat a-while to thee.
low and far a-bove, There my heart is ev-er light-est; In the spot I fond-ly love.

REFRAIN.

Dear old Wa-wa-yan-da, how I love thy shores With their fringing forests, where the wild bird soars;

hill en-cir-cled pict-ure, full of charm for me, Ev-er glad the mo-ment I may turn to thee.

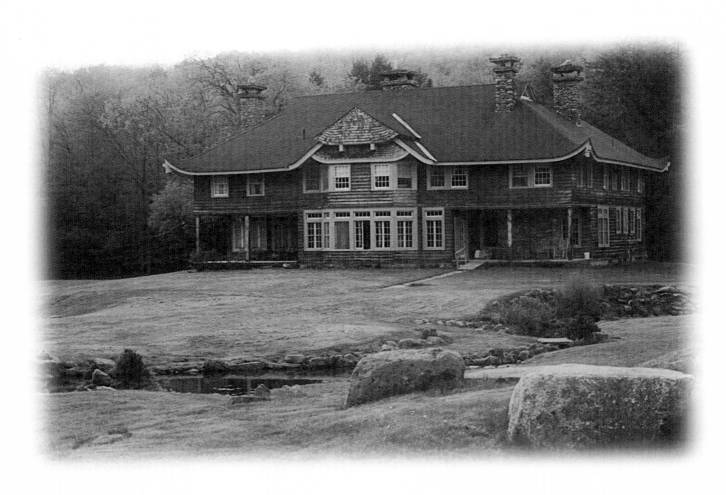

"Grey Lodge" on the East Branch of the Neversink.

Chapter 7

The '80s: Loss and Opportunity

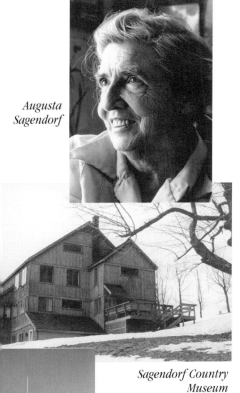

*Augusta
Sagendorf*

*Sagendorf Country
Museum*

*Weather station and
Harold Merrill
Pavilion*

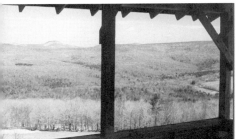

*Looking towards Frost Valley and Doubletop
Mountain from Merrill Pavilion*

The '80s began optimistically enough. Summer camp was thriving. The Environmental Education Program was growing steadily. Interest in conference facilities was invigorated with the opening of the renovated Straus Center, so much so that a full-time Conference Director was appointed. Frost Valley was welcoming an array of special interest groups to the beautiful Catskills all year round, and its programs reflected diversity and imagination.

The 1982 annual report was characteristically enthusiastic. Wrote Director of Camping Mike Ketcham: "We offered 25 different programs ranging from traditional resident camp to eight specialty camps (computer, soccer, gymnastics and more) and 21 adventure trips. More than 1,750 youth registered for summer programs in 1982. Campers came from 12 states and four continents. More than 150 skilled and dedicated men and women came together from 17 states and nine countries to form the summer staff."

There were new programs for campers with special needs: The Tokyo program continued for Japanese youngsters; a German language camp was offered in conjunction with the Steuben Society of Kingston; a group of blind cyclists enjoyed a tandem bike ride around Lake Champlain in a joint adventure with the New York Association for the Blind; asthmatic and developmentally disabled children had camping opportunities as did 160 disadvantaged youth from Newark, assisted, as always, with help from Victoria Foundation and Turrell Fund.

More than 12,000 people visited Frost Valley through the conference program, coordinated by new Director of Conferencing John Paul Thomas. Program income represented 32 percent of Frost Valley's budget. Not far behind in revenue and participation was the Environmental Education Program, which served 130 school groups and 8,000 students in 1982. Forty-five programs and activities were offered, including visits to the newest Frost Valley facility, the Sagendorf Country Museum on Red Hill.

A treasure trove of tools, artifacts and relics of local history, the museum was the domain of Augusta Sagendorf. Frost Valley had purchased, removed and replaced her derelict house with a handsome three-story residence and museum, where "Gusty" entertained visitors with stories and songs accumulated over a lifetime in the Catskills. The museum and its curator -- often charming, sometimes crusty, but never boring -- provided campers and visitors with a rare glimpse of mountain ways fast disappearing.

The Florence & John Schumann Foundation supported the project. Foundation Director Harold "Hal" Merrill had fallen in love with the view from Red Hill, and had pledged to do what he could to preserve it for future generations. He died unexpectedly in 1979, and in 1982 a pavilion was erected on the property in his memory. It is the hiking destination of choice for many campers, who continue to marvel at the unspoiled Catskill vista.

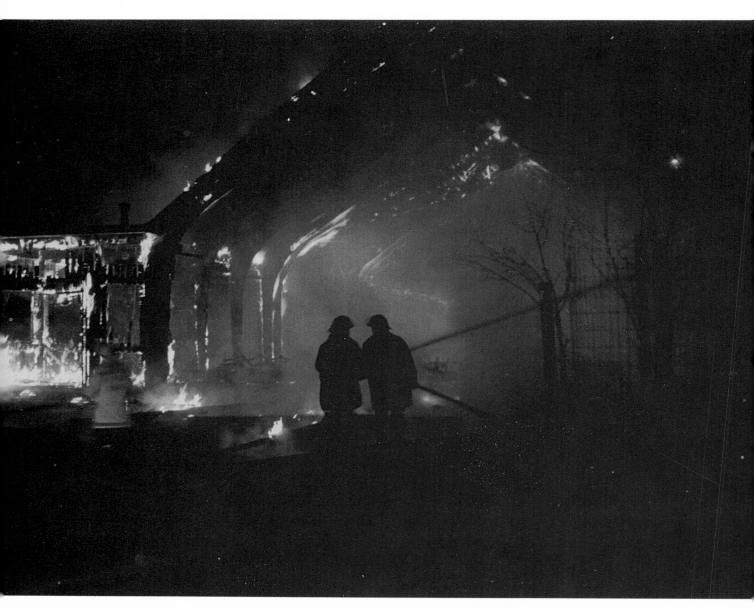

Frost Valley's view of the future looked rosy as 1982 drew to a close. Then came New Year's Eve.

Three-hundred guests and staff members had gathered to welcome 1983 with a celebration that included a traditional buffet in the boys' camp dining hall, Thomas Lodge. A staff show had been staged in Margetts Lodge and general merrymaking was taking place in various buildings. At 1:15 a.m., someone noticed flames and smoke issuing from Thomas Lodge. The fire truck housed in the little Frost Valley station was first on the scene. But even with water pumped from Biscuit Creek, and the arrival of volunteers and equipment from neighboring towns, the flames, believed started by an electrical problem, could not be quelled. By daybreak there was almost nothing left of the structure that had been the hub of camp activity for 24 years. A wooden plaque bearing the "Build Strong" credo was itself reduced to ashes. But a sign that had been erected just two years earlier, dedicating the Wawayanda Dining Hall to Frost Valley trustee H. Emerson Thomas, was salvaged. It would come to symbolize the determination to rebuild, to establish a new landmark bearing the Thomas name.

The disastrous fire proved to be a catalyst for major physical and organizational changes at Frost Valley. The loss of Thomas Lodge required the expansion of McLain Lodge, the summer dining hall at the

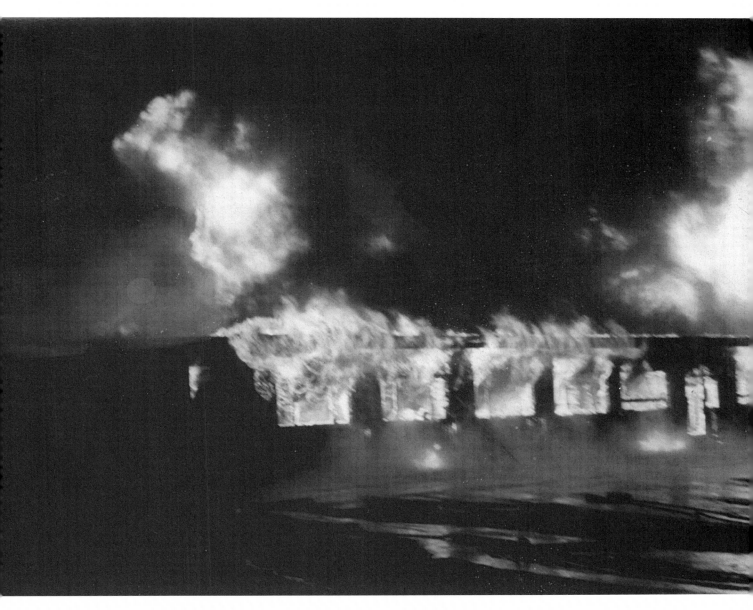

girls' Camp Hird, which had to serve both boys and girls (and all school groups, conference participants and visitors) for the next four years. The shared experience helped spur the idea of co-ed camping, which was adopted in 1983 with the designation of Camp Wawayanda as the summer home for younger boys and girls, and Camp Henry Hird the quarters for older campers. This facilitated age-appropriate programming and more normal socialization. That first year, the reorganization was administrative and programmatic; in 1984, campers were physically moved into the age-based camps.

The change did not come without some resistance from veteran staff and alumni, however. Terry Murray, Director of Camping from 1982 to 1987, said the opposition was more about the loss of the single-sex camping tradition than the idea of gender mixing. The campers took to the change almost immediately, though. "It made sense," said Murray, "and it reflected what was going on in camps across the country."

An equally significant outcome of the fire was the opportunity to create a new focal point for Frost Valley, one that would not only be its heart and soul, but its conscience as well. The new Thomas Lodge would mirror the institution's concerns for health and the environment, demonstrating real-world examples of energy conservation, resource recovery and wellness concepts. It would also serve as a model for future campus construction, which would employ similar innovations in design and operation.

The new dining hall was designed by Todd Schmidt of the architectural firm of Schmidt Copeland Parker Stevens of Cleveland. Schmidt had known Halbe and Jane Brown from his school days when he spent summers as a camper, counselor and staff member at the Youngstown Y's Camp Fitch. Schmidt's firm had since developed an international reputation in the design of environmental, outdoor and recreational facilities. At Frost Valley, Schmidt supported a master plan for the layout and design of several new buildings, as well as renovations to the Castle, Hayden and Margetts Lodges, the Straus Center and the administration building. His designs incorporated elements of the original structures and so maintained the feel and integrity of the Forstmann estate.

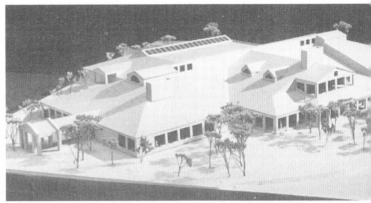

Architectural model of the proposed H. Emerson Thomas Lodge; below, completed lodge in 1986

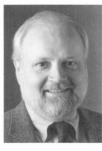

Architect Todd Schmidt

The $1.8 million dollar, 30,000-square-foot Thomas Lodge would accommodate 700 people in four dining halls. Like the old lodge but twice the size, the main hall would feature vaulted ceilings and a fireplace. But the building would also have skylights to allow some pas-

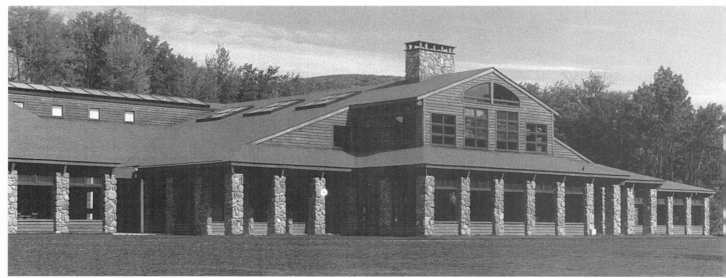

sive solar heating; energy efficient windows; super-insulation and water-saving fixtures. Built into the plans for future use were a refrigerated locker to store food waste for more efficient disposal, and infrastructure for a wood gasification plant that could utilize home-grown fuel and save as much as two-thirds on the cost of conventional oil heat. About 500 yards away from the dining hall, a 235,000-gallon steel tank reservoir was erected and a six-inch water line installed to the dining hall.

Project Director Chuck White, a state-certified building inspector and a member of the local planning board, supervised construction of the new facility, and of the renovations to McLain Lodge. At McLain, new food preparation and storage space was added, and an interior staircase installed linking the multi-purpose Conover English Room on the lower level with the upstairs dining room (later named for trustee Joseph Partenheimer). For the next four summers, McLain Lodge was a beehive of activity, as valiant kitchen staff essentially turned out six meals a day. With campers headed to and from the dining hall all day long, the path between Camps Wawayanda and Hird became so congested that the grounds staff widened it, some said to Interstate proportions. Thus it was given the nickname "Route 284."

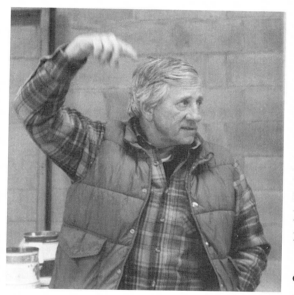

Chuck White, Thomas Lodge Project Director

The new Thomas Lodge took longer than anticipated to complete as board members and development staff undertook a concerted effort to raise the necessary funds. But by the fall of 1986, the facility was nearly finished and it was time to celebrate. Although the kitchen was not quite operational (meals for celebrants that October weekend had to be prepared at McLain and trucked to Thomas Lodge), the three-day event featured square dancing, cider making, hayrides and a dedication ceremony attended by, among others, 225 Indian Guide fathers and sons from Montclair. The singing troupe "Up With People" provided suitably vibrant musical fare. Solon Cousins, National Executive of the YMCA of America, was the guest speaker at the ceremony rededicating the lodge to H. Emerson Thomas, former mayor of Westfield, N.J., former chairman of the New Jersey YMCA, and an active Frost Valley trustee.

Individual rooms in the lodge were also dedicated to John Ben Snow, who helped develop the Woolworth department store chain; Louis Plansoen, a Newark leather company founder; Henry Balkan Day, a New Jersey businessman and father of Corbin Day, Frost Valley trustee and treasurer; and to James C. Kellogg III, former chairman of the Boards of the New York Stock Exchange and the New York-New

Woody English 1910-1996

One man can make a difference. That's what Woodruff J. "Woody" English proved time and again in 37 years as a Frost Valley Trustee. During his long tenure as Chairman of the Board, Woody English guided Frost Valley with wisdom, compassion, and spiritual strength. He gave generously of his time and energy, and encouraged many others to do the same. A partner in the New Jersey law firm of McCarter and English, Woody had served as President of the Newark YMCA, and as a tireless member of the International, Executive and Student Work Committees of the YMCA National Council. Frost Valley's expansion from a summer camp for boys to a year-round, far-reaching institution serving people of every age, creed, gender and nationality is due in large measure to the leadership of Woody English. In 1985, Frost Valley's Environmental Education Program was named in his honor.

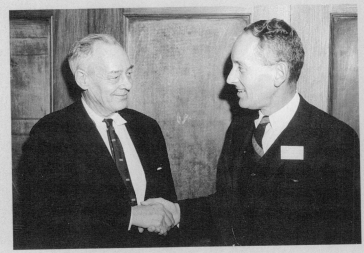

Walter Margetts and Woody English

Jersey Port Authority, and father of James Kellogg IV, President of Frost Valley.

Lounges in the new dining hall were named for Woodruff J. English and Judge Harry W. Lindeman. English had been a member of the Frost Valley board since 1959 and had served as President for many years. Credited with providing stability and guidance to the organization during its transition and growth years, "Woody" was also past President of the Newark YMCA, with a special interest in international work. In 1985, Frost Valley's Environmental Education Program was also named in his honor.

Harry Lindeman, a juvenile court judge in Essex County, N.J., had a lifelong interest in youth work and organized camping. He was a trustee of the Turrell Fund, which helped disadvantaged children attend Frost Valley. In 1979, a walking trail at the Straus Conference Center was also named for Judge Lindeman.

In 1987, carillons were installed at Thomas Lodge. They were a gift from Dr. Lowell Johnson, a businessman, leader and patron of many service organizations including the American Heart Association, for which he acted as National Chairman. Dr. Johnson was a friend of Dr. Jerome Wolff, an eye surgeon and Frost Valley board member who had helped spur the development of the

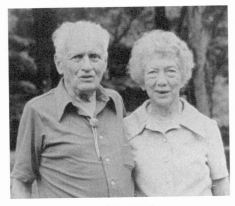

Harry and Em Lindeman

Howard E. Quirk, 1924-1994

He was a minister and a counselor; a raconteur and an enter-tainer; a chauffeur and a witty tour guide. Above all, Howard E. Quirk was passionate about people, the people whose futures he brightened as executive director of Newark's Victoria Foundation; the people whose eyes he opened on his famous "vertical tours" of St. John the Divine Cathedral in New York; the people whose lives were touched by his short but very sweet association with Frost Valley. In the five years before his death in 1994, Howard became the "heartbeat of Frost Valley:" He was a trustee, a full-time volun-teer at the Montclair office, director of the Endowment Fund and liaison with the Tokyo-Frost Valley YMCA Partnership Program. In 1998, Quirk Lodge, with its energy- and environmentally-conscious innovations, was named for the spirited man whose commitment to this place and its mission will long be remembered.

A meeting/classroom in Quirk Lodge was named Victoria Hall for the foundation Howard Quirk directed for 21 years.

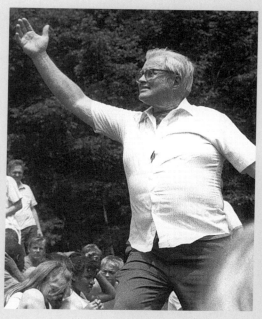

Howard E. Quirk

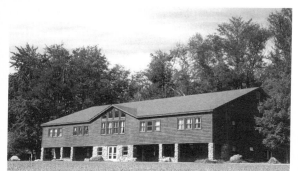

Hussey Lodge

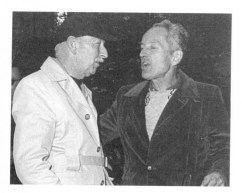

Fred Hussey and Woody English

Gottscho Dialysis Center and camp wellness programs.

On a parallel track with development of the new dining hall was an attempt to establish village lodges to replace aging camp cabins. First proposed in 1982, the lodges were in response to the need for more comfortable and efficient accommodations for year-round use by school groups and organizations. In 1984, Frost Valley accepted the largest sin-gle cash gift in its history to that point, a $300,000 grant from the Aeroflex Foundation, to build a prototype lodge in memory of Fred Hussey.

Hussey had, 30 years earlier, purchased the Camp Wawayanda property in Andover, N.J., setting in motion the camp's move to Frost Valley. Both Fred Hussey and his wife Nell had served as Frost Valley trustees, and upon his death, she chose to support the construction of a new lodge to symbolize her husband's interest in the facility's growth as a year-round service center and retreat.

Utilizing principles conceived and promoted by the Institute for Man & Science in Rensselaerville, N.Y., Hussey Lodge featured post-and-beam construction, wall and roof panels with high insulation factors, passive solar components, efficient windows, low-flow fix-tures and gas heat, chosen because of concerns over the safety of buried fuel oil tanks. Handicapped accessible, it could be used by special populations visiting Frost Valley. Hussey Lodge was dedicated in 1986.

The two-story, 13-bedroom lodge to sleep 70 people was envisioned as comfortably accommodating an entire "village" of campers, as well as off-season families. But it became apparent that the one-size-fits-all concept wasn't especially workable, and designers began to plan the first "cluster" of smaller, more flexible lodges. Scott, Neversink and Snow Lodges were designed like duplexes, with four rooms and 20 bunks which could be connected, or not, depending on need. These three lodges were built during the late 1980s and were dedicated in 1990. Staff quarters and meeting rooms were incorporated in the next group of lodges to be built – Bodman, Day and Kellogg. The last three to be constructed – Hyde & Watson, Quirk and Kresge – were twice as large as the preceding six and have become known as "super lodges," each accommodating as many as 40 campers or guests. The newest, year-round lodges have composting toilets, fireplaces and large meeting rooms, setting a standard that has been replicated at several camps across the country. Quirk was built into a hillside for energy saving purposes, and features solar panels.

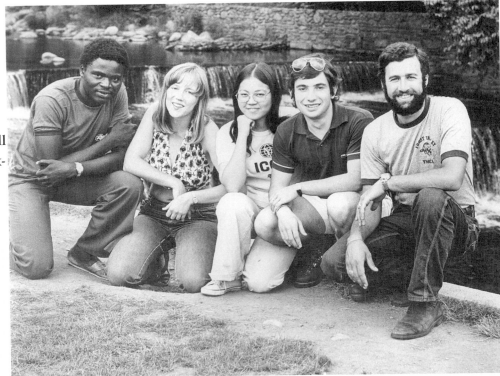

International counselors, left to right, unknown from Africa, Gudrun Mellberg, Wai Kwan Wong, Jean-Louis Lalanne, Bassem El-Hibri, 1985

These projects had not made the leap off the drawing board as Frost Valley celebrated the 100th anniversary of YMCA camping in 1984-85. The first observance of this milestone took place in October of 1984, when Halbe Brown co-chaired an international gathering of YMCA representatives in Estes Park, Colorado. Several Frost Valley staff members also participated. The following summer, campers celebrated with a birthday banquet and a Centennial Campfire, lit with a candle brought back from the Colorado event. A time capsule, holding wishes for the future penned by campers and counselors, was subsequently buried within the stonework at the east end of Thomas Lodge, to be opened 50 years hence, in 2035. Camper Barbara Scott, great-granddaughter of Wawayanda founder Charles R. Scott, led the

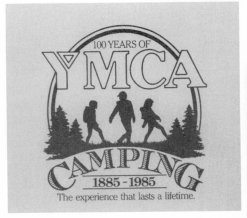

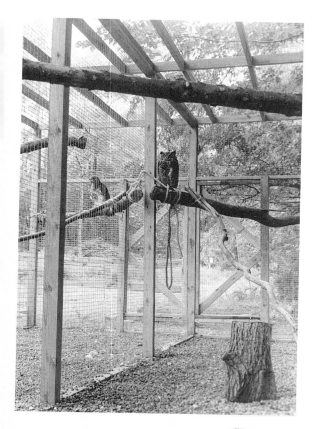

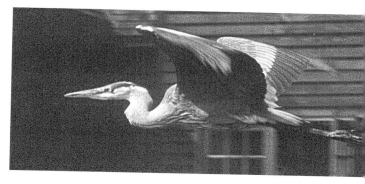

Susan Scherf, Raptor Center Coordinator, maintains the center as an important learning resource, a shelter for vulnerable creatures, and one of the most popular sites on campus, proving that, in the fertile Frost Valley environment, there will always be an emerging idea to explore, a new path to chart, a fresh opportunity to seize.

And there will always be room for a few more guests at the table.

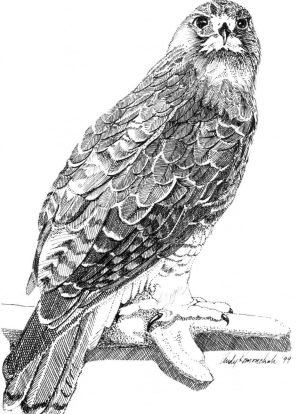

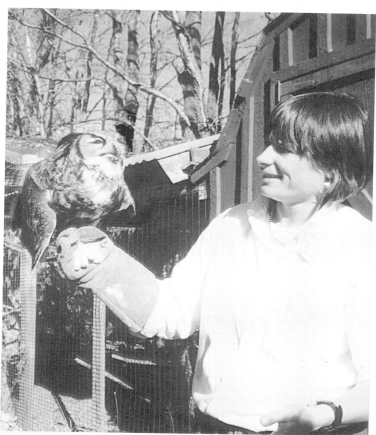

Raqptor Center Coordinator, Susan Scherf, with one of her guests

The living laboratories of forest and stream

Sometimes, Jim Marion can't believe how far Frost Valley's Environmental Education Program has come. He remembers the days in the late '70s, when he and the small education staff would skip from training sessions for teachers, to field workshops for kids, to dining room detail, setting mealtime tables for visiting groups, washing dishes, mopping floors. "Somedays we'd throw off our aprons and go out and teach a class or lead a cross-country ski tour," he chuckles.

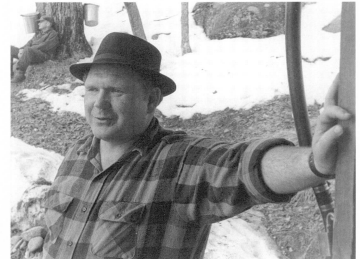

Jim Marion

As the program caught on, the staff grew, more revenue was generated, and the menu of program offerings expanded. Then, in 1983, a chance encounter with Peter Murdoch of the U.S. Geological Survey, who was taking a water sample from a stream on the property, led to an affiliation that brought original research into the classroom.

Frost Valley's involvement in a major long-term study on the effects of acid rain on mountain environments added an exciting new dimension to the Environmental Education Program, and supplied researchers with important data. The USGS sent Jim Marion to Louisiana for training so that Frost Valley could be an official acid rain study site, part of the National Atmospheric Deposition Network. It was the only cooperative venture between the USGS and a non-profit organization among the 19 "sensitive area" study sites being examined nationwide. The Frost Valley site held particular significance because of its location within the New York City Watershed, feeding a reservoir system that supplies water to nine million people.

Through the efforts of the USGS and the U.S. Environmental Protection Agency, a lab was set up in a former darkroom where Marion and biologist Claudia Swain tested water samples collected from Biscuit Brook. They checked for pH levels, conductivity, nitrates and sulphates. They monitored stream flows during storms, and took snow samples in the dead of winter. They sent pails of acid rain to the University of Illinois at Champagne-Urbana for comprehensive analysis. Eventually, they could tell where a storm had come from by the acidity level of the samples. During one serious gully washer that originated in the Ohio Valley with its coal-burning power plants, the

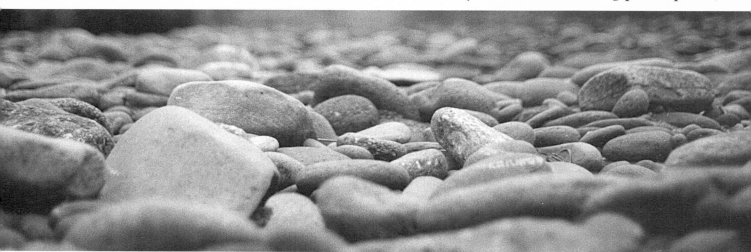

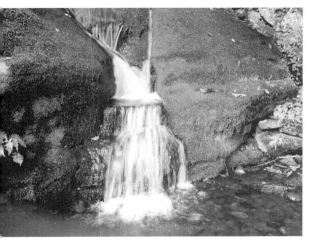

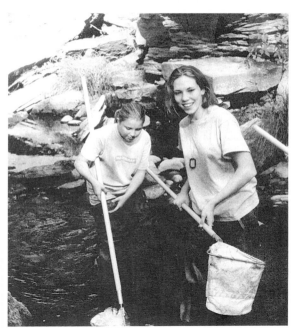

precipitation in pristine Frost Valley registered at 4.2; balanced pH is around 7. "That's more acidic than Coca-Cola. We were making sulfuric acid up there," Marion recalls.

That's a comparison his Environmental Education students could appreciate. "This was groundbreaking stuff. It was good science, and an excellent teaching tool," Marion said.

The successful collaboration with the USGS led to more long-term studies in the 1990s on the role of nitrogen on the

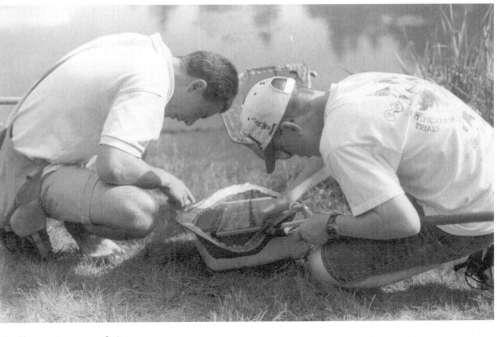

acidification of soils, and of the effects of forest harvesting on water resources. The multi-faceted project is taking place at three sites prepared by the Frost Valley Forest Management team. One plot has been clear cut, another has had 40 percent of its timber harvested, and the third remains undisturbed.

Researchers from the USGS, the State University of New York College of Environmental Science and Forestry, Syracuse University, the Institute of Ecosystem Studies, Rensselaer Polytechnic Institute and Vassar College are studying stream and soil chemistry, sediment transport, and nitrification rates over several years at the three sites. The objectives are to shed new light on the effects of forest harvesting on nitrogen and chemical processes, the implications for water quality and stream life, and the impacts of atmospheric deposition on climate change.

In 1997, Frost Valley was selected as one of three Forest Demonstration Sites within New York City's Catskill Watershed. Under the auspices of the Watershed Agricultural Council's Forestry Program, the site is intend-

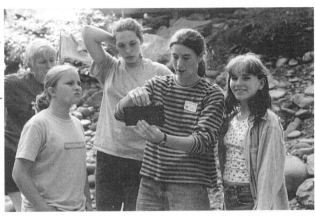

ed to show beneficial logging and management practices. Partners include the New York City Department of Environmental Protection, the U.S. Forest Service, Cornell University and the College of Environmental Science and Forestry at Syracuse.

An ambitious 100-year study of flora, fauna and ecological systems will make all of Frost Valley a living laboratory starting in 2001. Students, educators, researchers and concerned volunteers will be asked to help monitor ecological change at various sites over the coming century. Like the preceding 30 years of Frost Valley Environmental Education, it is science – and history – in the making.

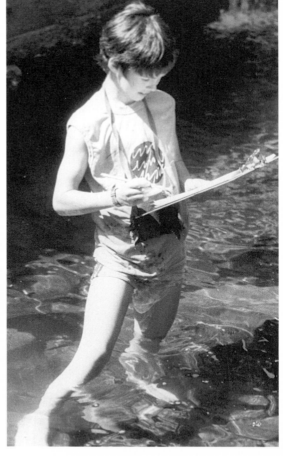

Environmental and ecological issues studies are only part of a multifaceted outdoor education program. Frost Valley's 25 environmental educators teach over 50 different courses for schools to choose from, allowing the students an experience which complements and enhances their lessons back in the classroom. "Academic learning, is always placed in a clearly practical context", stated Kris Henker, the Director of Environmental Education. "Students learn and apply basic geometry while using a compass, or geology by discussing the origins of the Catskill Mountains. They study current issues of land, forest and water management while learning about the taxonomy of trees to exploring the New York City watershed." Scientific discovery in an outdoor setting, along with scientific research enhances each learning experience. Frost Valley is a unique experience. Challenging, educational, yet always exciting for students, it can leave them with an indelible impression that will last a lifetime.

reunite with other families who've been doing the same thing for five, ten or 25 years.

Many staff members who make those reunions possible have been at Frost Valley for the same amount of time. Conference Director John Paul Thomas coordinated Family Camp activities (and gatherings of groups as varied as Green Nation, Newark Boys Choir, church groups and senior citizen clubs) from 1982 to 1992. He returned in 1999 to continue that role. The conference program has grown to include themed and holiday gatherings all year 'round. Tradition and possibility have always been equal and opposite motivating forces at Frost Valley. They merge seamlessly in the Centennial Plan for the Future, developed by the board of trustees under Chairman Paul Guenther. The plan invites readers to consider these ideas:

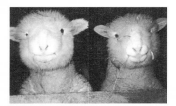

Some special friends at the Farm

The Frost Valley Educational Farm an innovative and far-reaching education program will provide school children, families and groups the opportunity to live, work, and learn together on our 582-acre farm. The farm program will feature year-round Residential opportunities teaching current "best-use" agricultural practices and traditional skills of early Catskill lifestyles through hands-on experiences. The

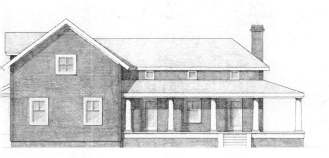

Frost Valley Educational Farm residence

farm's lodging, dining and educational workspaces will emphasize community living and outdoor classrooms will offer seasonal agricultural experiences.

The Halbe and Jane Brown Pavilion is planned as a centrally located facility that will provide a four-season check-in/check-out space for campers, schools and weekend groups. The Pavilion will provide a weather-protected area for sports activities and will include a large stone fireplace for inclement weather "campfires", making it possible to ensure that everyone receives a Frost Valley camp experience, "rain or shine."

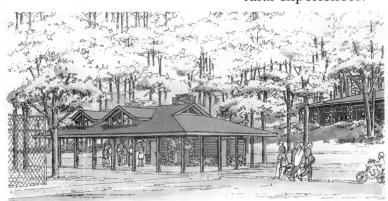

Cabin Renovations As Frost Valley moves forward in developing a modern campus with energy efficient lodges, the 30 original summer camp cabins, now outdated and inefficient, must be addressed. Several years ago the construction crew renovated two of these cabins with insulation, energy efficient windows, new heating, new beds and the addition of a covered porch as both a space for gathering and a place to keep wet clothes and shoes out of the cabin. By renovating and winterizing the remaining cabins we will be creating affordable year-round use and 100 additional beds at the same time.

Wellness Center The current Frost Valley health center, a refurbished 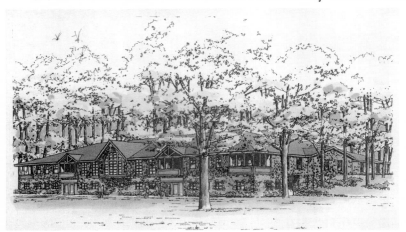 farmhouse, was intended for seasonal operation only when it began 27 years ago. At that time the first hemodialysis center in an outdoor setting was established at Frost Valley YMCA 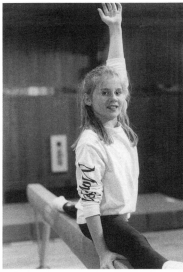 with a unique partnership between the Ruth Carole Gottscho Foundation, Montefiore Hospital and Frost Valley. This innovative program continues to provide mainstreamed resident camp experiences for 50 to 60 medically challenged children every summer. Since 1974 however, Frost Valley has become a year-round operation serving over 32,000 residential guests annually. The new Wellness Center is possible because of the long-term successful partnership with Montefiore Hospital and is planned to serve as a training and conference facility where children and families can learn to manage debilitating illnesses such as asthma, diabetes and renal failure. Montefiore Hospital will provide the medical personnel and Frost Valley will provide the location, facilities and mission-based program services. At the same time, the Wellness Center will provide new space for our health center and emergency services.

The Forstmann Castle Center for the Arts and Humanities

The historic Forstmann Castle continues to be the architectural centerpiece of our main campus. Extensive restorations of this 12-bedroom landmark building are necessary and continue as funds are received. An increasing interest in implementing an arts and humanities program at Frost Valley supports the need to remodel the ground floor as studio, meeting and lecture space. Scholars, artists, and musicians "in residence" could provide the resources for the presentation of writer's lectures, fine arts classes, and an expansion to musical events and concerts as part of a year-round arts and humanities program expanding educational and life enhancing opportunities for campers, families, and students as well as our community neighbors.

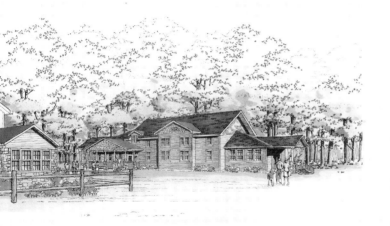

The Mitchell Lodge at The Straus

Center When Frost Valley helped establish the Wellness philosophy throughout the camping movement in the 1970s, much of this program was developed at the Straus Center, former home of Gladys Guggenheim Straus, a proponent of Wellness throughout her life. Today the Straus Center provides outstanding educational and retreat experiences for adults and families and is the primary site for Frost Valley's much-heralded Adult Education and Elderhostel programs. Families find that the secluded setting for annual

reunions provides the occasion to reconnect and renew. While the Straus Center is currently limited to an overnight capacity of 22 guests, the new lodge will increase capacity to 40. Plans

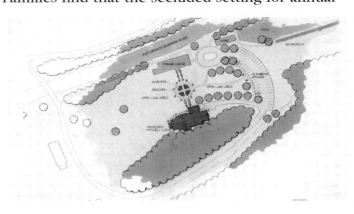

for the new lodge include handicapped accessible sleeping areas, a small kitchen, and much-needed classroom space.

The YMCA Board of Trustees has created a path to lead us into our second century of service to youth and families. They may seem ambitious plans, but no one – at least no one who knows Frost Valley and its Director, Halbe Brown – is prepared to discount them. "I could not have imagined then where Frost Valley would be today, but I'm not surprised," says Mike Ketcham who was on the staff in one capacity or another for 15 years beginning in 1971. "Halbe has always been innovative, he latches onto opportunity and he surrounds himself with good people."

Known by some as the "Mayor" of Frost Valley, Brown has been at the helm of this adventurous ship since 1966. It was his openness to new ideas that led to the highly successful environmental education program; his compassion that prompted Frost Valley to take on the challenge of providing dialysis for young renal patients; his aesthetic sense that pushed for beautiful – not just ordinary – camp buildings. And it was his vision that saw great potential in disaster.

Peter Swain had just been hired as a cross country ski instructor in late 1982 when fire destroyed Thomas Hall, the boys camp dining hall. "It was New Year's Day. I went up there at 5 in the morning, wondering if I'd just lost my job," he remembers. "I was standing in the smoke next to Halbe, listening to #10 cans explode, when I heard him say, 'This is an opportunity. We will rebuild.' That's when I understood there was a mission behind the place."

A mission that has not been derailed, despite changing tastes, interests and mores; despite setbacks like fires and floods; despite changing personnel and personalities. "We've always been flexible, not hesitant to try something new, or to back away if something didn't work," says James Kellogg. As a Frost Valley trustee for 30 years, and President for the past 15, he has seen the organization weather tough times and bounce back stronger than ever. Recalled Kellogg, "The gas crisis of the 1970s, for example, was a real worry. We had to do more busing since people couldn't get the gas to drive their kids to camp. But state funding for environmental education gave us a new revenue stream that allowed us to raise money not to fund deficits, but to build buildings."

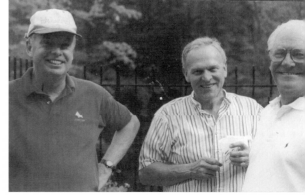

At a Neversink Society reception (left to right): Paul Guenther, Board Chairman, Halbe Brown, Executive Director and Fenn Putman, Treasurer of the Frost Valley YMCA Board of Trustees.

Kellogg is among committed board members who have ably kept Frost Valley's fiscal house in order so that its underlying mission – building strong kids and strong families – might survive.

Indeed, the Wawayanda/Frost Valley experience has for several generations changed minds, attitudes and lives. A great many people have spent years committed to the place, and to promoting the core values of honesty, caring, respect, and responsibility. "The cast of characters here has been a bit out of the ordinary, because relatively few people would devote their lives to a place like this, where they're not making a lot of money," says Roy Scutro, who has been involved with Frost Valley since the 1960s. "They are fundamentally like-minded folks, genuinely trying to do the right thing."

"There are a couple hundred of us who literally grew up here," says Al Filreis. "We knew nothing else but this place in the summer." Filreis was a camper from 1964 to 1970, then a counselor, then program director, and finally Camp Director of Wawayanda and of Hird before his "retirement" from Frost Valley in 1985 to become a professor of English at the University of Pennsylvania. Now, he brings his family up every summer, and recently joined the Frost Valley Board of Trustees as its first at-large member, representing a large and growing roster of former campers and staffers with lifetime commitments to the place and its mission. The Alumni Association, formed in 1987, has about 1,000 members who reminisce on a Frost Valley website, volunteer time and services to the organization, and contribute

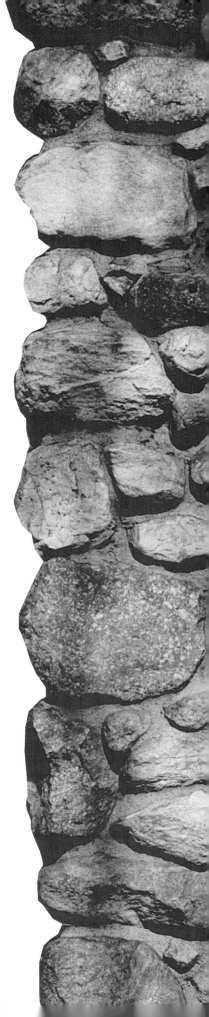

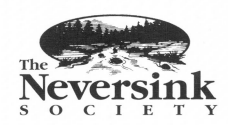

The Neversink
SOCIETY

*Like a river...the many friends who make up The Neversink Society provide
the strong current of experience and support which keeps us on course.
These are the men and women who have lived our history and are truly
dedicated to maintaining the vision of Frost Valley's future.*

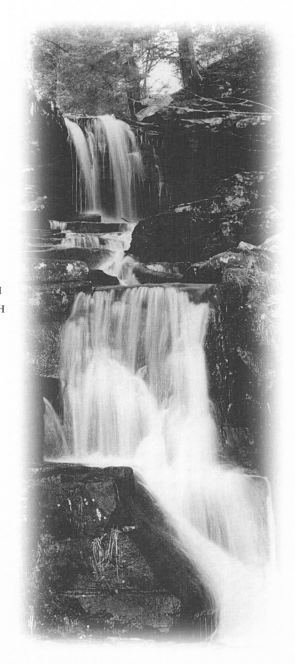

DAVID AND GAIL BAIRD
THOMAS AND THERESA BERRY
PAUL AND CARLENE BOLLERMAN
HALBE AND JANE BROWN
VERN AND BETTY CARNAHAN
ALBERT AND VERA CHRONE
JOHN W. DOUGLAS
MARGARET B. DUNGAN
STEVEN AND SUSAN EISENHAUER
BARTON C. ENGLISH
N. CONOVER AND ELEANOR ENGLISH
WOODRUFF J. AND CAROLYN ENGLISH
WILLIAM AND MARTHA FARNAN
AL FILREIS
STANLEY I. AND CAROL GARNETT, II
ROGER H. GILMAN
EVA GOTTSCHO
PAUL AND DIANE GUENTHER
DAVID AND MAUREEN HAIGHT, JR.
CHARLOTTE R. HAINES
ROBERT B. HAINES
WILLIAM AND PAT HAMILTON
JOHN AND KATHY HASKIN
DRS. GEORGE AND HELENE HILL

J. MAURITS AND KATE HUDIG
DAWN A. HUEBNER
HIRLEY KAY AND NORMAN GURI
JAMES C. AND GAIL KELLOGG
JOHN AND JODY KETCHAM
MICHAEL AND LOLLY KETCHA
ELIZABETH M. KOMLINE
CHARLES AND MARIE KREME
W. THOMAS AND DONNA MARG
WILLIAM AND BETTY MITCHE
MERRILL AND ELIZABETH OLES
JOSEPH AND LEILA PARTENHEIM
HOWARD AND BARBARA QUIR
THOMAS AND ELEANORE RICCIA
ROBERT L. ROOKE
MICHAEL AND MARGARET SCHI
ROSE AND SAL SENATORE
HALE AND FRANCES H. SEYMO
DONALD AND MARGARET SHERM
PETER AND CLAUDIA SWAIN
H. EMERSON THOMAS
EDMUND R. AND ELSIE TOME
JIM AND BOBBI VAUGHAN
DR. JEROME M. WOLFF

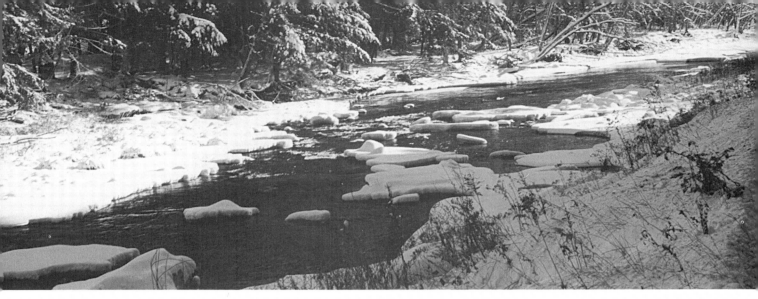

The future of Frost Valley is in your hands.

We invite you to join The Neversink Society, a special group of supporters who believe in the mission and vision of Frost Valley YMCA and who want to ensure that the Frost Valley heritage is continued for future generations. Designed to recognize contributions that build the long-range financial stability of Frost Valley, The Neversink Society honors supporters who make a significant gift to the Frost Valley Endowment Fund or who include Frost Valley in their estate plans. Such gifts may offer income and estate tax advantages that will enable you to provide much more security for both your family and Frost Valley than you ever dreamed possible.

You can qualify for The Neversink Society by....

- Including the Frost Valley YMCA Endowment Fund in your Will.

- Creating a Charitable Remainder Unitrust or an Annuity Trust, a Charitable Gift Annuity, Short Term Trust, Life Estate, or Bank Deposit that eventually directs all or a portion of the principal to the Frost Valley YMCA Endowment Fund.

- Naming the Frost Valley YMCA Endowment Fund as a primary or secondary beneficiary of an insurance policy.

- Making an outright gift of cash, stock, property, insurance, or an individual fractional interest to the Frost Valley YMCA Endowment Fund.

Recognizing Society Members

Names of Neversink Society members are engraved on a plaque that graces the entrance to Frost Valley's Edmund R. Tomb Administration Center. In addition, a special Neversink Society recognition dinner is held annually.

'What we have done for ourselves alone dies with us; what we have done for others and the world remains and is immortal'

Albert Pike

COMMEMORATIVE & RECOGNITION PLAQUES - BUILDINGS

The Tomb Administration Building and Historical Center
In Memory of Edmund R. Tomb

The Forstmann Castle The Friends of the Castle Endowment Fund
guided by Clara Hasbrouck

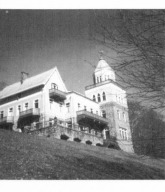

Major Gifts by
 Theodore Forstmann
Dr. Jerome M. Wolff
Robert B. Haines
William and Marion Nicholson
E.J. Grassmann Trust
The John Ben Snow Memorial Trust
F.M. Kirby Foundation, Inc.
Union Foundation

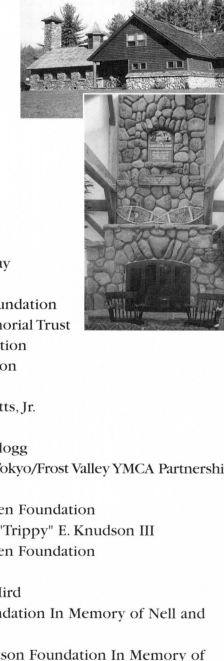

Lodges and Special Use Buildings

Bodman Lodge	Given by The Bodman Foundation
Day Lodge	In Honor of Clementine Corbin Day
Kellogg Lodge	In Honor of Elizabeth I. Kellogg
Scott Lodge	Funded by the Charles Hayden Foundation
Snow Lodge	Given by The John Ben Snow Memorial Trust
Neversink Lodge	Funded by The Day Family Foundation
	The Hyde and Watson Foundation
	The E.J. Grassmann Trust
Margetts Lodge	In Honor of Walter T. Margetts, Jr.
Turrell Hall in Margetts Lodge	Given by The Turrell Fund
Betty Kellogg Library	In Honor of Elizabeth I. Kellogg
Friendship House	Given in celebration of The Tokyo/Frost Valley YMCA Partnership
Tatsuo Honma Culture Sharing Center	In Honor of Tatsuo Honma
Hayden Lodge	Given by The Charles Hayden Foundation
Hayden Lodge Meeting Room	Given in Memory of Harry "Trippy" E. Knudson III
Hayden Observatory	Given by The Charles Hayden Foundation
Overlook at the Hayden Observatory	In Memory of Ritt Kellogg
Hird Lodge	Given by Henry and Rose Hird
Hussey Lodge	Given by The Aeroflex Foundation In Memory of Nell and Frederick Hussey
Hyde & Watson Lodge	Given by The Hyde and Watson Foundation In Memory of Lillia Babbitt Hyde and John Jay and Eliza Jane Watson
Kresge Lodge	Given by The Kresge Foundation
McLain Lodge and Out Trip	Given by Evelyn Bull McLain
Partenheimer Hall	In Honor of Joseph E. Partenheimer
Pigeon Brook Lodge	Named for Pidgeon Brook
Biscuit Lodge	Named for Biscuit Brook

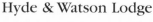

Ricciardi Cabin — Given by the Ricciardi Family
The Joy White Treatment Center — Dedicated in Honor of Joy White's years of service
Ruth Carole Gottscho Dialysis Center — Established by Eva Gottscho in Memory of Her Daughter - A partnership between The Gottscho Foundation, Montefiore Hospital and Frost Valley YMCA

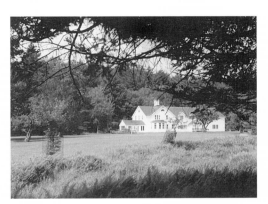

The Straus Wellness Center — In recognition of Roger Williams Straus and Gladys Guggenheim Straus

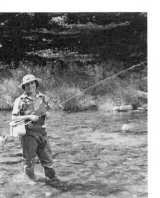

Bedrooms
   The Percy Chubb Room
   The Hayden Foundation Room
   The E.J. Grassman Trust Room
   The Knistrom Room
   The Clara Morthland Room
   The Mary Candace Seymour Room
   The Thompson Room
   The Helen Geyer Room
   The Gladys Straus Guggenheim Room
   The Florence Straus Hart Room
   The Gladys & Roger Williams Straus Room

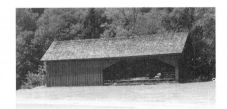

Public Rooms
   Lindeman Hall
   The Day Room - Solarium
   The Dodge Hall
   The Victoria Dining Room

Thomas Dining Hall — Dedicated in Honor of H. Emerson Thomas
Plansoen Room - In Memory of Louis M. Plansoen
Woodruff J. English Lounge - In Memory of Woodruff J. English
The Day Room - In Memory of Henry Balkan Day
The Kellogg Room - Given in Memory of James Crane Kellogg III
John Ben Snow Room - In Memory of John Ben Snow
Joseph C. Cornwall Room - In Honor of Joseph C. Cornwall
Lindeman Lounge - Given in Memory of Harry W. Lindeman by The Turrell Fund
R. Fenn Putman Entrance Hall - In Honor of R. Fenn Putman
Robert L. Rooke Entrance Hall - In Memory of Robert L. Rooke
Dr. Donald White Weather Station - In Honor of Dr. Donald White
The Carillon of Bells - Given by Lowell F. Johnson

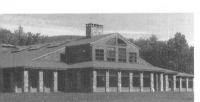

The Streamside Classroom — In Partnership with the United States Geological Survey, the NYC Department of Environmental Protection and the NYS Department of Environmental Conservation

| Howard E. Quirk Lodge | Given in Memory of Howard E. Quirk by his Family and Friends. |
| Victoria Hall | Given by The Victoria Foundation In Memory of Howard E. Quirk |

The Roehm Technology Learning Center

Mr. and Mrs. Luther S. Roehm   Steve Roehm
S. Scott Roehm   Geoffrey C. Roehm
E.J. Grassmann Trust   Union Foundation
Environmental Systems Research Institute, Inc.
The Charles E. and Joy C. Pettinos Foundation

Resource Management Center

Made possible through the generosity of the following foundations:

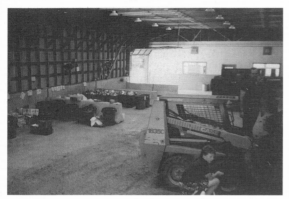

Florence and John Schumann Foundation
The Educational Foundation of America
John Ben Snow Memorial Trust
E.J. Grassmann Trust
Geraldine R. Dodge Foundation
The Hyde and Watson Foundation
F.M. Kirby Foundation
Warner-Lambert Foundation
Union Foundation

Frost Valley's Educational Farm

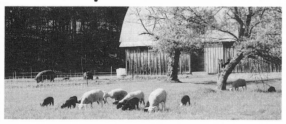

Made possible by the generosity of Peter Kellogg,
Paul B. Guenther, Kenneth L. Estabrook and James C. Kellogg

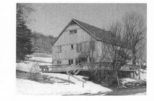

Sagendorf Museum   In Memory of Augusta 'Gustie' Sagendorf

Roadways and Trails

Turrell Way	Funded by The Turrell Fund
Carl Egner Memorial Nature Trail	A Tribute to a long-time friend, organizer and supporter of Camp Wawayanda.
Dr. Jerome M. Wolff Fitness Trail	Funded by Dr. Jerome M. Wolff
Lindeman Trail (Straus Center)	In Honor of Harry W. Lindeman
William and Bessie Erts Brook	In Loving Memory of the Erts Family
Schoonmaker Lane	In Honor of the Schoonmaker Family
Kellogg Road	In Honor of James C. Kellogg
Lake Cole	Named for Harry Cole - Forstmann Property Director

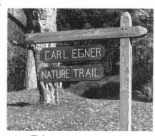

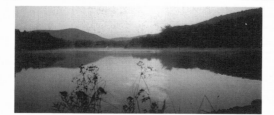

Harold Merrill Pavilion   In Memory of the Past Executive Director of the Schumann Foundation

Chapels/Meditation Sites

Poarch/Kilborne Outdoor Chapel Dedicated to Myron "Mike" Poarch and Charles T. Kilborne

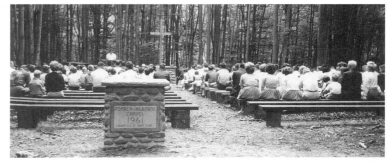

Ketcham Family Chapel In Loving Memory of Frank A. Ketcham and His Mother Laura W. Ketcham by Family and Friends

Memorial Garden and Reflection Pond

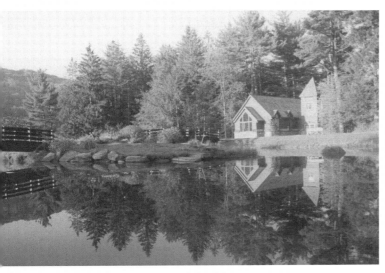

In Memory of:
Howard E. Quirk
Thomas Ricciardi
Hale Seymour
Francis Seymour
Jack Schloerb
Molly Ketcham
Trevor Haskin
Todd Schmidt
Margaret Haskin
Dr. William Morthland

Memorial Bench at Reflection Pond In Memory of wife and mother Peggy Hotz
Given by Laura, Waldo, Beckie and Dawn Hotz

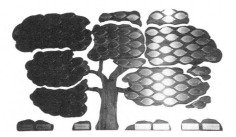

Giving Trees: Thomas Dining Hall
The Forstmann Castle
Ketcham Family Chapel

Campership Funds Victoria Foundation Turrell Fund
Sumitomo Foundation Alumni Fund for Camperships
Mark Selig Fund John Farnan Campership Fund
Rick McKay Scholarship Nash Fund

Commemorative Contributions
FOR
Frost Valley YMCA Camp Cabins

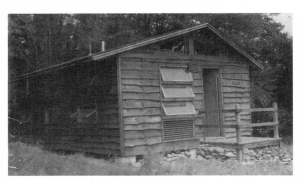

Bob's Cabin - In memory of Staff Sgt. Robert A. Hird by
Mr. and Mrs. Henry E. Hird 1958

In memory of Harold Sinley Buttenheim, Madison, NJ

Tom Hansen Memorial Cabin -Past District Governor of
Rotary International and VP of Bergen Co. YMCA
Given in Memory by Rotary Clubs

In Memory of Robert Haskell Cory, Chairman Bergen Co.
YMCA 1927-47, by Mrs. Robert Cory, 1959

Don G. and Constance W. Mitchell Foundation, 1960

Mr. and Mrs. Nestor J.H. MacDonald 1960

Evelyn Bull McLain 1961

Robert C. Crane, in memory of grandfather, Augustus S. Crane, 1961

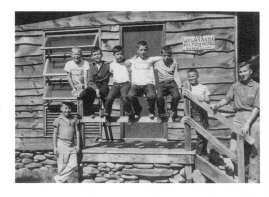

Mr. and Mrs. Earle B. Pierson

Mr. and Mrs. Judson T. Pierson	1958
Mr. and Mrs. Robert H. Rooke	1958
Mr. and Mrs. H. Emerson Thomas	1958
Mr. and Mrs. D. Harry Chandler	1958
Mr. and Mrs. Harry F. Cornwall	1961
Courier News, Plainfield	
Courier News, Plainfield	
Charles A. Frueauff Foundation, Inc.	1960
Charles A. Frueauff Foundation, Inc.	1960
Charles A. Frueauff Foundation, Inc.	1960
The Turrell Fund	1962

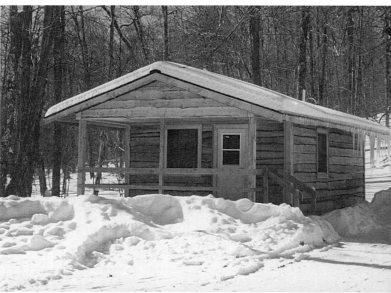

The Cabin Renovation Project will update existing year-round cabins and winterize others creating affordable year-round use and 100 additional beds at the same time. Our generation will be building the path for the next generation to walk upon. For additional information as to how you might help, please call the Frost Valley Development Office at 973-744-3488 or visit our web site at: *www.frostvalley.org.*

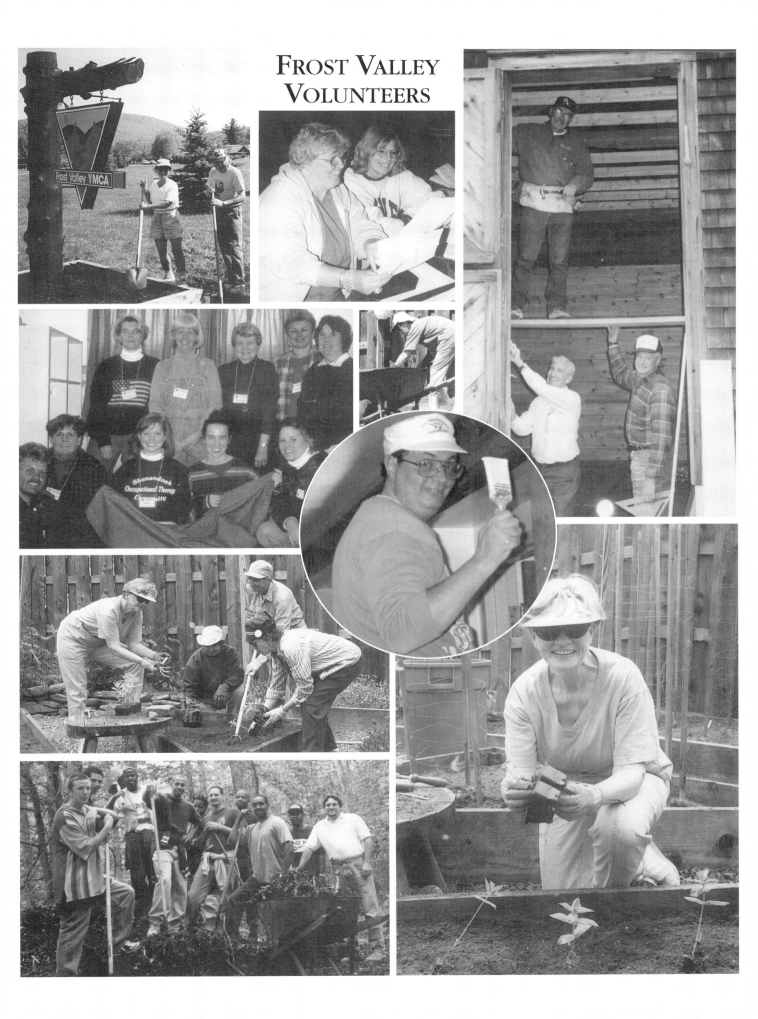

FROST VALLEY
VOLUNTEERS

INDEX

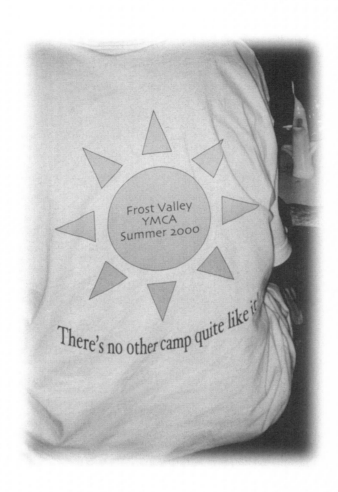